Mark Lauren is a certified Military Physical Training Specialist, Special Operations Combat Controller, triathlete, and champion Thai boxer. He has effectively prepared nearly a thousand trainees for the extreme demands of the most elite levels of the Special Operations community. As an experienced operator in mission planning and execution of airfield seizures, combat search & rescue, close air support, and reconnaissance & surveillance missions, he trained troops capable of immediate deployment into areas of forward combat operation by military freefall, static-line, all-terrain vehicles, overland, scuba, and other amphibious means.

Joshua Clark is the author of *Heart Like Water: Surviving Katrina and Life in its Disaster Zone*, a finalist for the National Book Critics Circle award. His work has appeared in many newspapers, magazines, and anthologies. He is also a certified personal trainer who has not set foot in a gym since Hurricane Katrina closed his fitness center; yet thanks to working on this book, he never stopped training, and is now in the best shape of his life.

Come say hi at MarkLauren.com

Other books from Light of New Orleans Publishing:

French Quarter Fiction: The Newest Stories of America's Oldest Bohemia
Southern Fried Divorce by Judy Conner
Back in America by Barry Gifford
How You Can Kill Al Qaeda (in 3 easy steps) by Howard Clark

Come see us at LightOfNewOrleans.com
to order signed books with free shipping.

YOU ARE YOUR OWN GYM

MARK LAUREN
and JOSHUA CLARK

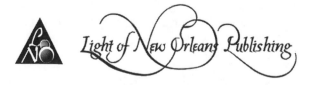

Light of New Orleans Publishing

Light of New Orleans Publishing, LLC
828 Royal Street, Suite 307
New Orleans, LA 70116 USA

Manufactured in the United States of America.

You Are Your Own Gym is intended for healthy adults, age eighteen and over. These exercises and programs are solely for educational and informational purposes. This information is in no way intended to be medical advice. Please consult a medical or health professional before you begin any new exercise or nutrition program, or if you have any questions or concerns about your health. The publisher and the authors do not assume any responsibility for your use of information in this book.

While the authors have made every effort to provide accurate Internet addresses at the time of publication, neither the publisher nor the authors assume any responsibility for errors, or for changes that occur after publication.

Back cover photograph by ZenShui/Frederic Cirou, courtesy of Getty Images.
Outdoor photographs of Mark Lauren: Laura Wong.
Exercise demonstration female model: Shea Garrison.

Library of Congress Cataloging-in-Publication Data

Lauren, Mark, 1972-
You are your own gym : the bible of bodyweight exercises / Mark Lauren and Joshua Clark.
p. cm.
ISBN 978-0-9714076-1-9 (alk. paper)
1. Bodybuilding. 2. Weight training. I. Clark, Joshua, 1975- II. Title.
GV546.6.W64L38 2010
613.7'13--dc22

2010003875

CONTENTS

In Memory of

Major William "Brian" Downs
Captain Jeremy J. Fresques "FS"
Captain Derek M. Argel "AL"
&
Staff Sergeant Casey J. Crate "CE"

Forward!

by John T. Carney Jr., Colonel USAF

*Colonel Carney has received numerous medals and awards for being at the forefront of
every mission involving our nation's Special Operations Forces since the mid-1970s.*

I can unequivocally state *You Are Your Own Gym* is a must read for anyone truly interested in their well-being. These principles, exercises, and programs will guide you to your highest fitness potential.

The credibility of all fitness authors comes from the men and women they have trained, typically movie stars and other famous persona. But the fitness of these celebrities is only achieved through countless hours spent one-on-one with a high-priced Hollywood trainer, while cooks are preparing their meals, housekeepers cleaning their homes, and assistants looking after their every need. Lauren's method, on the other hand, is for real men and women with real lives. *You Are Your Own Gym* separates itself from all other books by giving its readers the ability to train alone anywhere, any time, without the crutch of personal trainers and gyms.

In my book *No Room for Error*, I detail the involvement of U.S. Special Tactics Forces in operations ranging from the Iran hostage rescue to more recent ones in Afghanistan. The death-defying tasks that these troops accomplished and the hardships they endured were due to the incredible physical ability that matched their iron wills. Without it, their chances of success and survival would have been greatly compromised. It is only through the use of bodyweight exercises and sound training principles that these elite forces are able to maintain their astounding fitness at all times, regardless of time and equipment constraints.

The Special Operations community has developed the most effective and time efficient methods of training out of necessity. More than thirty years ago I was a fitness instructor at some of the same schools as Mark. I have seen the old and the new, and the methods of developing elite athletes have come a very long way, due in great part to Mark's leadership. Through the continuous application of the most up-to-date principles in sports physiology, attrition and injuries have been minimized while producing faster, stronger, and leaner soldiers.

This book comes to us at a time when, despite their best intentions, most people are too crunched for time and money to devote enough of either to attaining their fitness goals. In this age of information we are bombarded with incorrect advice, useless gadgets and pills, and pure hype. The methods outlined by Mark Lauren are proven and time tested. I know because I've seen his results. I've commanded the best of the best, and Mark's training has helped make them that way. Now he has honed his program into one for every man and woman.

In the 1970s Arnold Schwarzenegger showed the world the gym's potential, and it is said that he launched a thousand of them. Now it's time to harness the body's potential. This is the new fitness revolution.

1.

MISSION SUCCESS:
Lean, Strong, and Confident

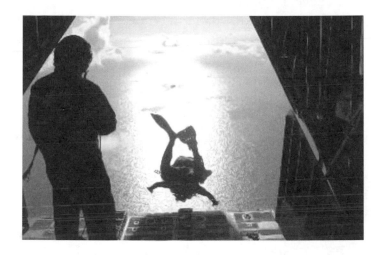

I WANT YOU TO UNDERSTAND, unlike many other fitness authors, I do not train movie stars, television celebrities, models, or other personalities whose livelihoods hinge on being fit. I train those whose lives do. For a decade I've used bodyweight exercises to create the leanest, strongest, most confident people of our civilization.

I honed the programs and myriad exercises in this book while preparing hundreds of trainees for the extreme demands of the most elite levels of the United States Special Operations community. I have spent years developing new training principles, and observing the results. A stellar record lead the top command to buy into my system. The military's most advanced forces—from Navy SEALs to Army Green Berets to Air Force Special Tactics Operators—use these exercises as the backbone to their strength training, and now I bring them to you. Now, for the first time, men and women outside SpecOps have the opportunity to reach the pinnacle of fitness, with an amazingly small sacrifice of your time. Clear, concise, and complete, I bring these exercises into your living room, bedroom, hotel room, garage, yard, office, wherever you like. They are for people of *all* athletic ability levels, tailored to suit the needs and lifestyles of today's busy women and men.

No book like this has existed before. Yet for thousands of years—from Ancient Greece's Olympic athletes to tomorrow's Special Operations forces—humanity's greatest physical specimens have *not* relied on fitness centers in their towns or dumbbells in their homes.

What if I told you that you already have the most advanced fitness machine ever created? Your own body. And what's so great about this fitness machine is that it's always there. It is the one and only thing you are never without. And now you're holding in your hand all the additional exercise equipment you'll ever need again. It's no longer necessary to spend hours and hours at a gym. In fact, you won't have to go to a gym at all. The time spent training, wherever you may be, will be minimal. Two hours per week. That's it. With these workouts you will not waste a single moment of your valued time using ineffective training methods. And no longer will you be able to use the #1 excuse for not training: "I don't have the time."

Whether you're a part-time fitness enthusiast, Olympic gymnast, bodybuilder, yogi, or someone who hasn't lifted anything but the groceries in years, my program will get you into the best shape of your life. You'll find an incomparable selection of the 111 most effective exercises to work any muscle you want, anywhere you want, for the rest of your life. With these clearly demonstrated and explained exercises you'll be able to construct your own training programs, catering to your needs and desires, that can be changed and modified in a virtually infinite amount of ways. Keeping your muscles guessing is how you keep them growing.

But for those who want the direction, I've laid out 10-week programs for all levels of fitness, programs that will lead to success where others have failed you before. You'll only workout 20 to 30 minutes a day, 4 or 5 times a week. I strongly recommend at least starting out with one of these programs. They combine the secrets to what made ancient warriors so strong, with the world's most effective and modern training principles.

These programs will increase the strength of important muscle groups needed in everyday living, keep your muscles and joints supple and flexible, improve the efficiency and capacity of the heart, lungs and other body organs, reduce susceptibility to common injuries as well as degenerative heart diseases, and reduce emotional and nervous tension. The benefits are never-ending. And success in your fitness program will inevitably lead to success in the other aspects of your life, both work and play.

This book can replace all other fitness programs in a person's life, or be used as a supplement to your regular program, as a way to change things up from the same ol' *borrrrrrring* routine in your fitness center, or even just to take on the road when you can't find a gym. Variety is the spice of life. Forget about doing the same sets and exercises day in and day out, maybe hitting the same treadmill every day, like a gerbil trapped in a wheel. And there's no need to change clothes, pack a gym bag, drive, park, find a locker, find an open machine... then, after a long, boring workout, do the whole process in reverse. You just start, whether at home, in your office, or a hotel room, and 20 – 30 minutes later you're finished.

You'll find no rhetorical filler in this book. No "before" photos of people pale and frowning with their glasses on, next to "after" photos of them tanned, smiling, flexing, and sucking their shaved and oiled tummies in. The proof has been before our eyes since man became man. In fact, even before that—why do you think monkeys are pound for pound stronger than humans? (Hint: It's not because they have Gold's Gym memberships.)

Do you really think that we evolved or were created to require machines in order to stay fit? It's lack of knowledge about your own body's potential that drives modern mankind's endless demand for useless fitness gimmicks. When in fact the solution to ultimate fitness is surprisingly simple. Though it's up to you to apply it. Free yourself from the dependency on gadgets, trainers, and common misconceptions. They are *all* crutches, keeping you from getting into the best shape possible. It's a call back to nature.

Your fitness should be dependent on nothing other than yourself.

2. HOW I GOT HERE

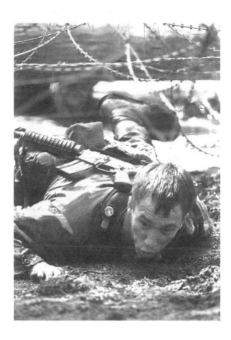

MY TEAMMATES WERE SPREAD throughout the length of the pool, ready to pull me up, because I was eventually going to pass out underwater. But for now, I stood in the water breathing and relaxing, getting ready to try to break the military's long-standing underwater record. I would need to swim underwater, on a single breath, for more than 116 meters. That's a good deal more than a football field, with the end zones included. Four months before, I could barely make 25 meters.

Everyone in the pool and on the deck was quiet, patiently waiting and watching me as I stood chest deep in the water. I knew this was going to suck, but I was committed. For the first time, I was alone in this, just me, without my team. It was surreal. I was calm, relaxed, aware. I was ready. My anxiety had evaporated. Without a thought, I took my last deep breath, went subsurface, and pushed off the pool wall.

You had to graduate one of the military's toughest selection courses to get on the record board, and with an 85% attrition rate, weekly evaluations, and an instructor staff dedicated to exploiting your weaknesses, graduation was far from a sure thing. In fact, it had already eluded me once.

My first time around, for 9 grueling weeks I fought tooth and nail to stay in the course. I'd be lying if I said quitting never tempted me. It tempted me every day, especially at the pool and in the mornings when a full night's rest felt like a 5-minute nap. Every weekend, my precious time off was spent learning to swim with fins and performing the various underwater exercises. At last, my final evaluation consisted of a 6-mile run in 42.5 minutes, 14 Pull Ups, 65 Push Ups, 12 Chin Ups, 70 Sit Ups, a 4000-meter fin swim in 80 minutes, and 7 torturous underwater confidence or "water-con" events. The fin swim was done with big thick rubber fins and booties that could push a large man with uniform and equipment through the water. You could not use your arms since it wouldn't be strategic for a team to swim ashore with arms flailing and splashing above the water. All calisthenics had to be done with perfect form. Each student's repetitions were counted and scrutinized by an instructor, and improperly executed reps weren't counted. Instructors shouted, "Didn't count, didn't count... Those didn't count... Your back is slouching... Not all the way up... Not all the way down!"

Staff Sergeant Pope counted my Sit Ups during the final evaluation, and of all the cadre, he was the most feared for his unreasonable treatment of trainees. "Those didn't count, Lauren. Your hands are too high up on your head," he said, shortly before failing me by 2 Sit Ups because of the position of my hands. That was all it took. On the last day of training, I got sent back to the junior class that was in week 1. My original class graduated 4 out of an initial 86. I walked back to the dorm as my team ran by in formation singing a jody about their last day. I seriously considered quitting.

But the last nine weeks had taught me something I would use for the rest of my life. A successful team was one that was made up of individuals that were able to set themselves aside. We were trained to set aside personal comfort for the common goal of the team. And that training applied as much to a team as it did an individual. Success is about you—and no one but you—letting go of everything that conflicts with your goal.

So I started over from scratch. Daily, we got smoked for hours doing exercises in the San Antonio summer sun, on top of the course's regularly scheduled workouts that consisted of a 60-minute run, 2 hours of cals, water-con, and an hour of finning. But it was always getting started in the morning that was the hardest.

On average, we did an extra 500 team Push Ups throughout the day, but really it didn't matter. We eventually learned that no matter how tired, stiff, and lethargic we felt, once we got warmed-up again, we were alright. Every time we entered or left the school house we had to do either 15 Pull Ups, 13 Chin Ups, 20 Dips, or 20 Chinese Push Ups. Once we each had to do 1000 team Push Ups without getting up except once for 5 minutes to use the latrine. For three and half hours, as a team, we did 5 Push Ups at a time, resting between sets by putting our butts in the air or slouching at the waist. 1000 Push Ups (+1 for teamwork) for having too much tape on our snorkels.

But bad as any of these smoke sessions ever were, the worst was always the pool. During the first few weeks of training, trainees would joke and chat on the way to the pool. By week 6, the bus rides were filled with silent dread. You could here a pin drop. It was the pool that caused the majority of the course's tremendous attrition rate. You could quit at any time. If you decide that it isn't for you, just say it: "I quit." In the middle of any event you could get out of the pool and go eat pizza in your room.

Monday through Friday we went to the pool, and trainees could only get out of the pool one of three ways: Successfully complete the events, quit, or pass out trying—in which case you would get pulled out just long enough to regain consciousness before going back in to accomplish the task, quit, or pass out again. Screwing up an event meant that you would have to do it again and each following attempt got harder and harder, especially events like equipment recovery—diving to the bottom of the pool, removing all our equipment and placing it in perfect order on the bottom, then putting it all on again before inspection—or knot-tying—we had to tie three different knots perfectly 12' underwater—that required you to tread water between dives. We learned to commit, stay down, and get through it the first time no matter how bad it hurt. It was all about being fully committed. Commitment equaled success.

This was INDOC—9 weeks of sucking it up for the team while 9 instructors tried to make as many of us quit as possible. My second time around, a team of 12 made it to the final evaluation and all passed but one. A teammate failed the 4000-meter fin. We would be going back to the pool one last time so he could take his re'eval. My time had come.

I remember sitting on the bus, regretting that I had mentioned challenging the underwater record. I knew my teammates wouldn't let it slide, and before long, one called me out. "So you really want a shot at the record?" he asked. "You really gonna do it?" I wanted to break his nose, but instead choked out a "Yeah." I was committed, and he laughed at my upcoming misery. But he was right, it was time to walk the walk.

As our teammate took his re'eval finning for 78 minutes, I sat on the side of the pool relaxing and breathing. I had a daunting task ahead of me. The discomfort of not breathing is overwhelming, and I knew that once I started, I wasn't going to be above the surface of that water until my teammates pulled me out unconscious. I had committed myself to breaking one hell of a record. A1C Switzer, a 6' 3" collegiate swimmer, had set the record at 116 meters. When I first got into the course, I remember saying that of all the records, the underwater record was the most impressive. A 116-meter underwater to a trainee that is struggling with 25-meter underwaters seems god-like, and here I was, four months later, at the end of my second class, getting ready to challenge it.

With my feet on the gunnel, I sounded off: "Ready to enter the water, Sergeant!"

"Enter the water!" replied the instructor.

"Entering the water, Sergeant!"

I stood at the side of the pool breathing and relaxing for a few more minutes as my teammates waited for me, ready to pull me out when the time came. I took my last deep breath, went subsurface, and pushed off the wall.

I was utterly alone. After two months of nonstop teamwork, I could suddenly neither see nor hear anyone or anything but myself. My total focus was on my stroke and relax-

YOU ARE YOUR OWN GYM

ing. Stroke, glide, relax... Stroke, glide, relax... until finally my body started cursing me for not breathing. But my goal was in place. And my comfort would not interfere.

At the 50-meter point, just as the discomfort was starting to seriously crank up, I had a fleeting thought of standing up out of the water and laughing it off, but I couldn't do it. Your mind always looks for a way out when things really get difficult. Relaxing, maintaining good form, and pressing on when the body and mind beg you to do otherwise tests your resolve. *Stroke, glide, relax... Stroke, glide, relax...* Tension, panic, anxiety make massive withdrawals on a very limited and precious oxygen supply. I had to stay relaxed long enough to get through the worst of it. *Stroke, glide, relax... Stroke, glide, relax...* Eventually the discomfort eases once your brain and other body tissues are starved of oxygen and you become hypoxic. It seemed an eternity before I got to that point, but eventually the lights dimmed, my peripherals vanished, things weren't so bad after all, and the tunnel got smaller and smaller until...

I woke up on the other side of the pool, pale and blue-lipped. "Did I get it?" I mumbled. I wasn't able to remember swimming the whole length of the pool, nor passing out just as I reached the wall. I had started sinking at that point, and my teammates jumped in and yanked me out. I began breathing again. I had just set the new record—one I still hold—at 133 meters, after swimming subsurface, on one breath, for two minutes and twenty-three seconds.

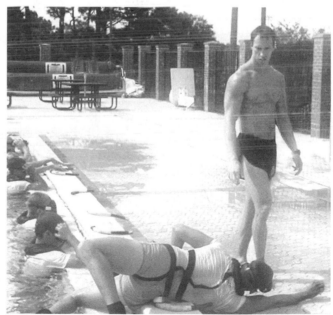

I feel your pain. Years later, I became the instructor.

I'LL ADMIT, MY FIRST FORAY INTO FITNESS was driven by nothing more than body image. I was 13, a scrawny, shy kid, and I wanted to do something about it. I set out to change my physique into one I could show off with pride. I had no access to weights, so I did Push Ups and Sit Ups in my bedroom before dinner. Until I could do 75 non-stop Push Ups and 600 Sit Ups. Then I did more. I became a stronger version of myself in every way, and confidence in all I did soared, including winning regional high school bodybuilding titles.

Many years later, at the Pararescue & Combat Control Indoctrination Course, if we weren't running, swimming, or holding our breath, we were performing some type of bodyweight exercise. Training lasted from 5 am to 6 pm, Monday through Saturday, and by the end of the nine week course there was only a small handful of us remaining, less than 15%. The high rate of attrition was largely due to overtraining. Though the training mentality of that time was amazingly effective at shattering young men's perceived limitations, it was not ideal for optimal fitness.

Once on team, at the 22nd Special Tactics Squadron, I continued to use bodyweight exercises to keep myself physically fit and able to meet the extreme demands of airfield seizures, combat search & rescue, and reconnaissance & surveillance missions.

Five days before September 11, I left my team to become a full-time Military Physical Training Specialist. It became my responsibility to prepare trainees to meet the demands of immediate deployment into areas of forward combat operation.

After Sep 11th, the demand for SpecOps soldiers went through the roof. The career field needed numbers. The days of graduating only 5 - 15% of the original class had to end. The cadre was forced to look at its training methods. We used to be old school: More is better—run the trainees into the dirt and make them hard, or get rid of them. Changing to "less is more" wasn't easy, but necessity forced us, and we were in the perfect environment to learn quickly what worked and what didn't. Every six weeks I got a new shipment of untrained recruits. Most came to me soft and weak. By the end of the course, they were lean, strong, and confident.

By applying the most up-to-date strength and conditioning principles and sports science, I was able to produce better results with only a fraction of the time and less injuries. I experimented with varied volume and intensity, day to day, week to week, and included sensible recovery and progression. I revamped the courses' physical training programs, and personally tailored these programs and diets to suit the individual needs of candidates, and then monitored their progress.

Amazingly, despite limited space, time, and equipment, as well as larger classes, I was able to cut the course's attrition rate by 40%. And in every class I taught, at least one of my students captured the coveted Army Special Forces Honor Graduate award. Quite simply, I built a training method superior to any other in developing muscular, lean, physically fit bodies as fast as possible. And now I share it with you.

Embrace the exercises and principles in this book and you will become fitter and stronger than you've ever been. It's in your hands, literally, starting right now.

3.

WHY BODYWEIGHT EXERCISES?

THE POPULARITY OF TRAINING EQUIPMENT, systems, and fad diets is mostly the result of marketing—not a genuine attempt to help a generally out-of-shape society reach higher levels of fitness and well-being. In this age, where our homes and gyms are cluttered with fitness gadgets, the simplest and most effective method for developing strength and losing fat has been largely overlooked—knowing how to train using nothing more than your body.

Even outside of SpecOps, the efficacy of bodyweight exercises has been proven time and again. Take, for example, Madonna, Bruce Lee, or the USSR's two-time Olympic gold medalist Alexeev—arguably the strongest man in the world in his time—who was the first to clean and jerk 500 pounds, or Dallas Cowboys running back Herschel Walker who gained more yards than anyone in professional football history (and had a body to match). They, and countless others, primarily used bodyweight exercises to attain their ultimate physique and fitness.

Most weight training exercises isolate only certain muscles, requiring a fairly small portion of your body's total muscle mass, unlike bodyweight exercises that incorporate many at once. These exercises have the added benefit of being much more demanding of core strength (*6-pack anyone?*) than exercises that require weights and machines.

Bodyweight exercises also use motions that keep you safe from the many chronic injuries, like joint problems, that come over time with weightlifting and other unnatural exercises which have little functional value in our daily lives. For an exercise or workout to be functional, it must resemble the event being trained for as closely as possible. The performance demands of the average person consist mainly of manipulating their own bodyweight throughout the day. So what could be more functional for developing better strength in day-to-day activities than bodyweight movements? But between couch potatoing and bench pressing—sitting on your butt and lying on your back—we've got a nation of functional weaklings. Seriously, when was the last time, outside of using gym benches or machines, that you exerted yourself while sitting or lying down? (*While you were alone, I mean. ;-)*)

For too long these exercises have gone largely unnoticed by popular culture. Other than running and swimming, most people haven't been raised to use their body alone for exercise. The exploding popularity of yoga and pilates is a great example of the worth of bodyweight movements, although these methods, when used alone, utterly lack a systematic approach to developing all-around fitness.

My program has the advantage of making you proficient at using the one thing that you are never without: Your body. You will develop greater strength, power, muscular and cardiovascular endurance, speed, balance, coordination, and flexibility. Combined with a good diet and consistency, it will reward you with continuous results, challenges, and much greater body control.

The workouts can be done anywhere, anytime, and without costly gym memberships or equipment. With that said, even for those that insist on lifting weights, these exercises are a valuable addition.

You will be training as Achilles did before battle on the shores of Troy, training as ancient warriors the world over knew was best, training as future SpecOps warriors will to meet their own foes. Why? Because it works.

MYTH:
BODYWEIGHT EXERCISES DON'T ALLOW YOU TO ADJUST THE DIFFICULTY OF AN EXERCISE

There's a common misperception out there that bodyweight exercise options are limited. Push Ups, Pull Ups, Sit Ups—and not much else. *Hmmmm...* Did I mention that there's over 111 different exercises in this book? And that's not including their variations. The fact is there's a far wider array of exercises in this book than there are machines in any gym in the world.

Other people think it's impossible to work certain muscle groups with bodyweight exercises. Wrong again. Every single muscle group, and some you didn't know existed can be worked without weights—from getting rid of a pencil neck to using your shin muscles to round out your calves.

The only limiting factor with bodyweight exercises is your creativity. Every weightlifting motion can be mimicked, made harder or easier, with your own bodyweight. And unlike those machines in the gym, there are seemingly infinite ways to vary any of my exercises, keeping your muscles guessing and growing for the rest of your life.

For example, I detail Push Ups that even a 600-pound man (or 70 year-old woman, for that matter) could do. And then there's ones, like the Planche Push Up, most professional bodybuilders won't be able to execute without lots of practice. My 10-week program actually comes with specific workouts laid out for different ability groups, so that everyone will be challenged equally.

Here are the four simple ways of changing the difficulty of an exercise without adding weight:

- Increase or decrease the amount of leverage.
- Perform an exercise on an unstable platform.
- Use pauses at the beginning, end, and/or middle of a movement.
- Turn an exercise into a single limb movement.

Again, let's take the Push Up, a standard exercise that works your chest, shoulders, triceps, abs, obliques, and lower back (unlike benching which only works half of these). If you do Push Ups standing up with your hands against a wall a couple of feet in front of you, the exercise is pretty easy. Then try them with your hands on an elevated surface, like the edge of a bureau or windowsill. The lower the surface you use—a desk, a couch, a coffee table, telephone books—the harder it gets. Putting your hands on the floor, like a standard Push Up, is harder. If we put our feet on the coffee table and our hands on the ground, the exercise becomes significantly more difficult. This is using *leverage* to increase the exercise's difficulty.

To make the exercise still harder we could place our hands on one or two balls, like a basketball. Now we're using an *unstable surface*.

Still harder would be to do basketball Push Ups with pauses at the bottom. Still not hard enough? Try doing them one-handed on the floor. Then one-handed with your feet on the couch. Then on an unstable surface. Then with pauses... You get the idea.

And this is only a simple example that can be repeated with many of my exercises. You'll see the possibilities are endless.

So there you have it: We've gone from one variation of an exercise, that probably *everyone* reading this book can do, to a more difficult variation that probably *no one* reading this book can do right off the bat. The difficulty of bodyweight exercises can be tailored to suit the needs of virtually anyone. You have total control of the resistance.

4.   WHY STRENGTH TRAINING?
(or *Why Cardio Is a Waste of Your Time*)

WHETHER YOU WANT TO LOSE FAT, gain muscle, or do both, strength training should be the core of your conditioning. Aerobic activity, on the other hand, is inefficient and ineffective no matter your goal.

It is a myth that doing prolonged steady state training—usually maintaining a target heart rate for 30 to 60 minutes—like aerobics or "cardio" is the best way to burn calories and achieve cardiovascular health. Ever plod along on a treadmill that tells you the number of calories burned? You might go 45 minutes before you hit 300 calories. Well, guess what? That's 300 *total* calories burned in that time, and not 300 calories above what your baseline metabolism would have burned anyway, even while at rest. That's the reason the exercise machine asks your weight: To calculate your baseline metabolic rate. The average male burns 105 calories at rest in 45 minutes. Those 195 extra calories that the exercise *actually* burned—only 195 calories more than if you had been taking a nap—can be undone by half a plain bagel in half a minute. And aerobic exercise typically spurns your appetite enough to more than offset those few actual calories burned.

Here's the skinny: One pound of fat can fuel the body for up to 10 hours of continuous activity. If we were so metabolically inefficient as to burn calories at the rate the exercise equipment advertises, we would never have survived for so long, and certainly not endured the hardship of the Ice Ages. The calories expended hunting and gathering would have caused us to die of starvation long before we ever found a Wooly Mammoth. By today's standards, we would hardly have enough metabolic economy to survive a trip to the super market, let alone hump it across enemy lines for a week-long reconnaissance mission with 120 pounds of gear.

More bad news for aerobic activity: Whether it's running, cycling, or a step class, the main reason it gets easier the more you do it, is *not* because of improved cardiovascular conditioning, but because of improved economy of motion. For the most part, it doesn't get easier because of muscular endurance, but because your body is becoming more efficient at that particular movement. You require less strength and oxygen than you did before because your body's nervous system is adapting. Wasted movements are eliminated, necessary movements are refined, and muscles that don't need to be tensed are relaxed and eventually atrophied. This is why marathon runners will huff and puff if they cycle for the first time in years.

Aerobic training actually causes muscle *wasting* because the body is programmed to adapt to whatever demands we place on it. Long low-intensity aerobic training only requires the smallest and weakest, "slow-twitch" muscle fibers to fire off again and again. The other, stronger and larger, "fast-twitch" muscle fibers are not necessary for the task and become a burden to carry and supply with oxygen. The body has no demand for extra muscle beyond what is needed to perform a relatively easy movement over and over. So your body adapts by actually burning muscle.

The reason many people gain weight as they age, especially beginning in their 30s, is because they have less muscle than they had in their late teens and early twenties. As we age, our bodies naturally lose muscle, especially as we are less active in our lives. This muscle tissue loss results in a decreasing metabolic rate. And then, if you continue to eat like you did when you were younger... well, you'll slowly gain weight, pound by pound, month by month, year by year, until one day you look in the mirror and wonder, "What happened?" The key to eliminating accumulated body fat is regaining your youthful metabolism by regaining your muscle.

Muscle is the most metabolically expensive tissue we have: It takes between 50 and 100 calories a day just to keep one pound of muscle alive, for both men and women, even if you are completely inactive. An extra five pounds of muscle can burn up to 15,000 calories in a month—that's the equivalent of two pounds of fat. Muscle is the single greatest tool for weight loss. Increased muscle mass let's you lose weight with less attention paid to calorie counting and food selection.

But with consistent aerobic exercise, over time, you're far more likely to *burn* five pounds of muscle. That means your body will burn *at least* 250 *less* calories a day. And as your body becomes more efficient at running, that 195 calories you burn on the treadmill will decrease to about 125. So let's do the math: You burn 125 calories above your resting metabolic rate each day you do aerobic exercise. Then add the minimum 250 calories you do not burn due to muscle loss caused by this exercise. After all your huffing and puffing you are now 125 calories in the wrong direction!

THE ANSWER: INTERVAL STRENGTH TRAINING

Interval training is the repeated performance of high-intensity exercises, for set periods, followed by set periods of rest. Intervals can consist of any variety of movements with any variation of work and rest times. It burns far more calories and produces positive changes in body composition with much less time than aerobic training.

This is not only because of the muscle it builds, but also the effect it has on the metabolism *following* the workouts. Strength training gives your metabolism a boost far beyond the duration of the actual workout, for as long as 48 hours. In contrast, after aerobic training your metabolism returns to normal almost immediately. So with interval training we're not only building muscle, but we're also able to kick up our metabolism for the rest of the day—even when sleeping!

Many people believe aerobic activity strengthens their heart, and decreases the chance of things like coronary artery disease. Yet, after much research, even U.S. Air Force Cardiologist Dr. Kenneth Cooper—the very man who coined the term "aerobics"—now believes there is no correlation between aerobic performance and health, longevity, or protection against heart-disease.

On the other hand, aerobic activities do carry with them a great risk of injury. Most, even so-called "low impact" classes or activities like stationary cycling, are not necessarily low-force. And things like running are extremely high-force, damaging to your knees, hips and back. Aerobic dance is even worse. Sure, you'll hear the occasional genetic exception declare that they've never ever been injured doing these exercises. But overuse injuries are cumulative and often build undetected over years until it's too late, leading to a decrease or loss of mobility as you age, which, in turn, too often leads to a shortened lifespan.

Any effect you are seeking from aerobic activity can be achieved more safely and efficiently with high-intensity strength training. Remember, your cardiovascular system supports your muscular system, *not* the other way around. An elevated heart rate means nothing by itself. Being nervous before a full combat equipment nighttime High Altitude Low Opening (HALO) formation jump always sent my heart rate skyrocketing, but it didn't make my belt any looser. And even if you insisted on measuring the efficacy of an exercise by an increase in heart rate, I dare you to get it up higher than with my "Stappers."

So there we have it: Interval strength training is superior to aerobic activity in burning fat, as well as building strength, speed, power, and even cardiovascular endurance. All this in far less time than tedious "cardio" sessions.

Dr. Angelo Tremblay and his colleagues at the Physical Activities Sciences Laboratory, in Quebec, Canada, tested the popular belief that low-intensity, long-duration exercise is the most effective program for losing fat. They compared the impact of moderate-intensity aerobic exercise and high-intensity interval training on fat loss.

Skinfold measurements revealed that the interval training group lost more body fat. Moreover, when they took into account the fact that the interval training used less energy *during* the workouts, the fat loss was *9 times* more efficient in that program than in the aerobics program. In short, the interval training group got 9 times more fat-loss benefit for every calorie burned exercising. How can that be?

Because, after taking muscle biopsies, measuring muscle enzyme activity, and lipid utilization in the post exercise state, they found that high-intensity intermittent exercise caused more calories and fat to be burned *following* the workout. In addition, they found that appetite is suppressed more after intense intervals.

Throughout the book you'll find **Hooya!** boxes with information, facts, studies, and ideas. SEALs and Special Tactics Operators yell "*Hooya!*"—an American Indian war cry meaning "Give me more!"—when they drive through their personal comfort to achieve the seemingly unachievable.

Izumi Tabata and his partners at the National Institute of Fitness and Sports in Tokyo, Japan, compared the effects of moderate-intensity endurance and high-intensity interval training on maximal aerobic capacity—the best indicator of cardiorespiratory endurance. They conducted a six week study with two groups of randomly picked males.

Group 1 did one hour of steady state training five days a week. Group 2 did *only 4 minutes* of interval training five days a week. At the end of the six weeks, Group 1 had an increase in maximal aerobic capacity of 10% and Group 2 had an increase of 14%. Not only did the interval group have a 40% greater gain in aerobic capacity, they had an increase in strength of 28% percent, as opposed to the Steady state group which had no gains in strength. And all this with just *four minutes* of interval training a day.

Similar studies have confirmed that interval training produces higher gains in aerobic fitness, greater decreases in body fat, and gains in strength as opposed to the muscle wasting that occurs with much longer sessions of steady state training.

5. SO WHAT IS "FITNESS," ANYWAY?

SURPRISINGLY, THERE IS NO CLEARLY DEFINED, universally accepted standard for fitness. In the decade I spent honing military units assigned to carry out the most dangerous missions, it was always my experience that the individual with the best development in all areas of physical ability succeeds the best operationally. Similarly, it is diverse ability that makes us attractive.

Not to offend anyone, but I think most people would agree that a sprint athlete looks more attractive than a powerlifter, a ballet dancer better than a marathoner. The sprinter and the dancer have a higher level of fitness than the bodybuilder and marathoner. Their muscles tie together in a functional way. Most people would agree that it's the physiques with the most development across a spectrum of physical qualities that are most attractive, as opposed to those that have very limited usefulness. It is diversity in physical ability that is most useful and functional, not to mention beautiful. In contrast, those who are extremely developed in a certain area almost always have a weakness equivalent to their strength. The super fast, skinny runners lack strength, and the bulky bodybuilder types have little endurance.

So, my program develops the entire spectrum of physical skills: Muscular Strength, Muscular Endurance, Cardiovascular Endurance, Power, Speed, Coordination, Balance, and Flexibility. The degree to which you possess these eight physical qualities defines your level of fitness.

It is only by focusing on these seven skills, rather than appearance, that you will make your best gains, in ability, well-being, *and* in appearance. The washboard stomachs, big chests, round shoulders, and shirt-sleeve-stretching biceps of my men are testament to that, as are the toned legs, tight triceps and abs of the women I've trained.

MUSCULAR STRENGTH: Your ability to exert a force through a given distance. Muscular strength can be determined by the difficulty of an exercise that you are able to perform for a single repetition. For example, if Jane, with maximal effort, can perform one Classic Push

Up and Tarzan can perform a Handstand Push Up, then Tarzan has greater muscular strength.

POWER: The amount of force you can exert in a specific amount of time. Power = Work/Time. If Tarzan and Jane are both able to perform only one Pull Up with their maximal efforts, but Jane is able to perform that one Pull Up faster, then she has more power even though they have the same strength.

MUSCULAR ENDURANCE: How long you can exert a specific force. Jane and Tarzan could compare their muscular endurance by seeing who can hold the peak position of the Pull Up the longest.

CARDIOVASCULAR ENDURANCE: Your body's ability to supply working muscles with oxygen during prolonged activity. Jane and Tarzan challenge and improve their cardiovascular endurance by performing 200 non-stop Squats together.

SPEED: Your ability to rapidly and repeatedly execute a movement or series of movements. If Jane can do 45 lunges in 30 seconds and Tarzan can do only 25, then Jane has greater speed.

COORDINATION: Your ability to combine more than one movement to create a single, distinct movement. For example, performing a simple jump requires that you coordinate several movements. The bend at the waist, knees, and ankles and then the correct extension of those joints must all be combined into a single movement. Your ability to combine these movements, with the proper timing, into one movement determines your coordination, and in turn, how well you can do the exercise.

BALANCE: Your ability to maintain control of your body's center of gravity.

FLEXIBILITY: Your range of motion. If Jane, while doing a squat and using good form, can go down until her butt touches her heels, and Tarzan can only go until his thighs are parallel to the ground, then Jane has greater flexibility.

Simply put, fitness is the degree to which a person possesses these seven qualities.

Now, you may be thinking, "Okay great, now we know what fitness is, but what does that have to do with the real reason I bought this book?"

I know that most people are reading this book because they want to look and feel better, not to improve their balance, flexibility, and coordination. Herein lies a common mistake: Most programs put the cart before the horse. It is by focusing on the development of these seven skills, rather than appearance, that you will make your best gains, both in ability *and* in appearance. Form follows function. Well-being and healthy, attractive physiques are tied together, and they are best created through my program that develops all the qualities that make up fitness.

Naturally, those with the greatest all around level of fitness have always possessed the greatest ability to survive. And it only makes sense that we would evolve to find those with the greatest ability to survive the most attractive.

So how are all these levels of fitness developed? Through the use of short strength training sessions using bodyweight exercises and a sound nutritional plan.

6.

NUTRITION:
Back to Basics

I CAN JUST SEE IT: A trainee's reply to being told that they will, at a minimum, eat a mandatory three meals a day at the chow hall: "Excuse me Sergeant, this isn't going to work at all. You see, I'm on the grapefruit diet..."

There are too many different diet books out there, most advocating one extreme or another. Not only are many of these unhealthy, but folks just don't stick with them. How on earth are you supposed to apply some of these diets at a restaurant or dinner party? Stay away from fad diets and empty promises of magical formulas. Instead stick to the *fundamentals of healthy eating*—balancing quality sources of protein, carbohydrates and fats. Avoid the pitfalls of dieting and develop a lifetime of healthy eating habits that are in-line with your goals.

In our age of quick fixes and empty promises, sound and reliable eating principles seem to have been lost. Instead we're drowning in a sea of useless and unhealthy fad diets accompanied by continuously contradicting advice from so-called "experts." There is simply no magic pill or ground breaking new diet that can quickly and easily solve all your problems. The *only* reliable method of reaching and maintaining your long-term fitness goals is by understanding and consistently applying dietary fundamentals.

The value of a good diet cannot be overemphasized, and it's probably much easier to pull off than you expect. Understanding the basics and getting into a routine is simple. Many people just need to break some old habits and misconceptions. You do not have to be miserable, to eat well. The right diet should make you feel better, not worse.

Whether you are trying to gain muscle, loose fat, improve athletic ability, simply stay healthy, or all of the above, you *only* adjust your calorie intake according to your goals. The rest stays the same: Consistently perform short, intense, strength training sessions, and eat a balanced diet. No matter your goal, you should consistently strength train, try to get 7 – 8 hours of sleep a night, and you should eat frequent meals, maintaining an even flow of energy, leaving that afternoon slump at the door. Your eating habits won't be driven by hunger, and your cravings will be controlled. You're not a caveman anymore. You do not need to stuff your face, thus storing a bunch of fat for warmth, because there's a good possibility you won't find another Wooly Mammoth for a few days. Fat is your body's way of storing energy so you don't starve later. If your body gets used to eating several meals a day, it quickly learns there isn't any reason to store fat, because it knows there's no starvation period coming up. This means five or six small meals a day, every three hours or so. Don't worry, I'll show you how this is practical and easy.

Don't be surprised if you find information in this chapter that runs contrary to commonly held beliefs, the same beliefs that contribute to the runaway obesity rate in our society. First let's start with some basic definitions. Giving these a good read will be sure to correct any misconceptions you might have, and misconceptions are people's biggest hindrance to reaching their goals.

CALORIES

The amount of energy released when your body breaks down food. Proteins, carbohydrates, fats, and alcohol contain different amounts of calories per gram. Weight gain, weight loss, and weight maintenance is, to a large degree, but not exclusively, a matter of calories (energy) in vs. calories (energy) out. Somewhat oversimplified, excess calories are stored as fat, and a calorie deficit causes stored fat to be burned for energy.

WHAT YOU EAT vs. HOW MUCH YOU EAT

Among dieticians and fitness enthusiasts there is an ongoing, heated debate about what you eat vs. how much you eat.

Some claim weight control is simply a matter of what you eat. They believe if you eat the right foods in the right proportions, you'll be healthy. Eating the wrong things is what causes unhealthy cravings for excess calories. This is because bad foods can throw our hormones out of whack, feeling unsatisfied and under-nourished

On the other hand, the calories in vs. calories out folks believe that weight control is simply a matter of how many calories are eaten in relation to how many calories are burned, regardless of what the food sources are. Using this theory, a person maintaining a calorie deficit of 500 calories per day should loose one pound per week, since one pound of bodyweight is equivalent to 3500 calories (500 calories x 7 days = 3500 calories).

Which of these is right? They both are. But, even though it might sound funny, I have to say that the "what you eat people" are more correct. I know this both from science and countless trials. The proof is in the pudding.

Yes, you will lose weight by creating a continual calorie deficit, but if those limited calories are coming from mainly overly processed foods with little nutritional value, it will leave you feeling terrible and constantly craving food. Plus, such a diet will reap havoc on your hormones causing you to cannibalize muscle instead of burning fat. This is the diet that most people turn to and it is the reason why weight loss is rarely permanent.

As I will discuss shortly, the body's resting metabolic rate (RMR) is a key player in our ability to stay lean, and it is affected to a large degree by our body composition with muscle being our greatest calorie burning ally. With that said, it's important to place the emphasis on a positive change in body composition and not just weight loss. Loosing muscle weight is bad and counterproductive. Using the calories in vs. calories out theory alone, can at best give you a temporary fix. It's unrealistic and unhealthy to go through life following a diet that causes you to feel tired and hungry while your hormones run amuck.

Instead, use a combination of the two theories. It's just as unrealistic to expect people to always eat perfectly proportioned meals as it is to continually follow a restrictive diet without emphasis on nutritional value. Yes, it is true that consistently eating meals with the correct ratio of macronutrients will minimize excess cravings, but doing so is much easier said than done. For most of us, forever eating perfectly balanced meals at every sitting just isn't going to happen. We should strive for balanced meals, and if that's not possible, we should look to at least balance our macronutrients—carbs, fats, and proteins—throughout the day, if not in every single meal.

Hooya!

EVOLUTION AND THE DOMESTICATION OF PLANTS AND ANIMALS

Vegetables. Fruits. Nuts. Seeds. Meats. Eggs. Fish.
That's it.
For millions of years our ancestors survived purely from these 7 things. Typically, the women gathered the nuts, seeds, fruits, and vegetables while men hunted for meat. Together these food sources provided the necessary components of a complete diet that sustained healthy living. Climate, geography, and luck mainly determined how balanced these sources were. But remember, regardless of how much of each food they ate, these were the *only* foods available to our ancestors, so naturally our bodies have adapted to their consumption.

It wasn't until about ten thousand years ago, a blip in our time on Earth, with the cultivation of plants and domestication of animals, that large quantities of breads, potatoes, rice, pasta, and dairy became available. These relatively new sources of calories were the main reason our complex societies were able to develop, and our overabundance is to a large degree due to them.

However, for millions of years our bodies evolved on diets without any of these. The relatively miniscule time span since the domestication of plants and animals has not prepared us to live healthy lives with diets consisting of too many breads, pastas, rice, and potatoes. Yes, life expectancy has greatly increased in this time span, but this can be attributed not to new foods, but rather to man's no longer having to live life on-the-go while dealing with hunger, thirst, illness, injuries, extreme cold, and fighting dangerous animals with primitive tools.

So think of these new calories as little more than fillers. If you find yourself overwhelmed by nutritional definitions and rules, just ask yourself this: For millions of years before the domestication of plants and animals, what did we eat?

MACRONUTRIENTS

Macronutrients consist of proteins, fats, and carbohydrates. Contrary to common belief, each is a necessary part of a healthy and effective diet regardless of your goals. Some popular diets advocate cutting either fats or carbohydrates out of one's diet. At best, this only benefits you in the short term, since these diets are nearly impossible to maintain permanently. Each macronutrient plays a vital role in our health and well-being, and excluding any one of them will cause you to feel unsatisfied and tired.

Whether we are trying to shed body fat and gain lean muscle mass or just trying to bulk up, our goals are best met by eating a fair share of each of the macronutrients. Daily, we should aim to consume 1 - 1.5 grams of protein per pound of ideal bodyweight, with the rest of our calories coming from an even split of good carbs and fats.

CARBOHYDRATES

Each gram of carbohydrate contains 4 calories. Carbs are a key source of energy, especially for the brain. They include fruits, vegetables, pastas, grains, sugars, cereals, and rice. All carbs are made of sugars and classified as either simple or complex carbs based on the number of sugar units within a carb's molecules. All carbs are converted to glucose, a type of sugar, before they are absorbed into the bloodstream. Then they are either burned for energy or stored for later use.

Carbs are absorbed into the bloodstream at different rates. Highly glycemic carbs that absorb too rapidly into the bloodstream have several downfalls because of the strong insulin reaction that they produce. Insulin is an important hormone that regulates the body's blood sugar levels and storage of glucose as fat or glycogen (glucose that is stored in the liver and muscles).

SIMPLE AND COMPLEX CARBOHYDRATES & THE GLYCEMIC INDEX

Pasta, potatoes, oats, vegetables, and grains all contain complex carbs. Complex carbs must first be broken down into simple sugars and then those simple sugars have to be converted to glucose before they can be absorbed into the blood.

Simple carbs are found in foods such as fruit (fructose), dairy products (lactose), and table sugar (glucose).

Again, a carb's rate of absorption into the bloodstream produces a proportionally strong release of the hormone insulin. Rapid absorption of glucose causes rapid secretion of insulin. This in turn signals your body to store fat. And this is followed by fatigue and cravings for more carbs due to the blood's sudden depletion of glucose. Obviously, this isn't what we want. So the longer it takes for a carb to be broken down into glucose, the better.

However, it's not as simple as only eating complex carbs. For numerous reasons, many simple carbs actually absorb at a much slower rate than many complex carbs. Most fruits, for example, contain fiber that slows down the digestion process. Also, sugar that comes from fruit (fructose) and dairy (lactose) must first be converted to glucose before it can be absorbed into the blood, causing yet another slowdown in the digestion process. You will actually feel satisfied for longer by eating an apple versus an equal-sized bowl of pasta. Because even though pasta contains complex carbs, those carbs are still broken down into glucose faster than the apple's sugars.

To make all this a bit simpler, we can use a glycemic index to determine what carbs to eat. The glycemic index measures the rate of absorption of carbs. A carb that has a low glycemic index absorbs slowly (good), and a carb with high glycemic index absorbs rapidly (bad). For a comprehensive list of foods and their glycemic indices, see MarkLauren.com. You will find that many fruits and vegetables have a much lower glycemic index than grains and pastas.

Choosing your carbs doesn't stop there though. Carbs should also be chosen based on their nutritional value. The problem with foods such as table sugar isn't just their high glycemic index, it's also that they provide no vitamins, minerals, fiber, or good bacteria. Ideally, the carbs we eat should be as close to their original form as possible, such as whole pieces of fruit (not fruit juices), raw or steamed vegetables, dairy, and oats. Much of our obesity problem in Western civilization can be attributed to consuming massive amounts of carbs with high glycemic indices and little or no nutritional value. Many people, mistakenly, believe that they can eat whatever food they want as long as it's low in fat, regardless of the glycemic index, nutritional value, and caloric content. Everything from cookies, yogurts, sports bars, fruit juices, cereals, and sodas contain large amounts of table sugar that should be avoided.

Craving sweets from time to time is normal, but a diet with excessive sugar can cause these cravings to get out of control. Part of the problem is the insulin spike caused by these sugars. The insulin rids your blood of its glucose leaving you feeling tired and craving more glucose to replace the glucose that has been emptied out of your bloodstream. This creates a vicious circle.

The solution? Eat carbs with a low glycemic index. As much as possible, especially for those of you looking to shed body fat, get your carbs from whole pieces of fruit and raw or steamed vegetables, because they have the lowest glycemic index and contain valuable nutrients. The next best source is dairy and whole grain products.

FATS (Friendlies, not enemies!)

Don't believe the hype. Dietary fat is not the enemy of weight loss. And dietary fat does not automatically convert to body fat. Fat is vital not only for optimal performance and weight control, but it's absolutely necessary to sustain life.

Fats are calorie rich with 9 calories per gram versus 4 calories for protein and carbs. There are two types of dietary fat: Saturated and unsaturated.

Saturated fats tend to raise bad cholesterol and triglyceride levels and chances of heart disease. They are mainly derived from animal sources and foods containing hydrogenated oil—from margarine to muffins, fish sticks to potato chips, instant potatoes to popcorn, and too much of what you find at fast food chains.

Unsaturated fats tend to lower bad cholesterol and triglyceride levels and chances of heart disease. They come from plant sources such as nuts, seeds, non-hydrogenated vegetable oils, soy, olives, olive oil, flax seed oil, and fish.

Both types of fat provide us with added satiety, improved taste and texture, a great energy source, and slowed absorption of other nutrients. These are the major reasons why many low fat diets leave people tired and constantly craving more food. The satiety that you'll get from a little extra fat in your diet will allow you to comfortably eat less calories than you would without the fats.

Dietary fats even contribute to the regulation of the body's hormones. Research has shown that men who get less than 30% of their calories from fat produce 25% less testosterone than those who have more fat in their diets.

Fat should make up 25 - 35% of our total calorie intake. But be sure to consume mainly good, unsaturated fats. A small palmful of nuts and seeds, a bit of healthy oil on your salad, and eating plenty of fish will provide you with enough of the unsaturated fats. And those saturated fats you do eat should only come naturally from the dairy and meat you consume, not from foods such as French fries, butter, potato chips or other junk foods.

PROTEIN

The most important, but most commonly neglected macronutrient. Protein breaks down into amino acids, the building blocks used to repair and regenerate all cells of the body, including your muscles. Adequate protein intake is essential not only to maintain but grow muscle. Protein makes you feel full faster than fats or carbs, which is obviously beneficial if you're on a restrictive diet. It's got 4 calories a gram, and major sources include poultry, meat, fish, dairy products, soy, tofu, beans, and eggs.

A person trying to build muscle through resistance training needs to consume about 1.5 grams of protein for every pound of ideal bodyweight. People restricting their calorie intake for weight loss need to ensure that they still consume at least 1 gram of protein per pound of their ideal bodyweight and optimally 1.5 grams per pound, in order to prevent any loss of muscle while cutting fat. If you do the math, it's probably more protein than you're used to. For a 150 pound woman, that means consuming 150 - 225 grams of protein a day. But trust me, you'll see the difference once you re-prioritize your macronutrients like this. Protein should be the center of every meal. Choose your source of protein, then select the healthy carbs and fats you want to add to it (if needed). Keep in mind, even with 225 grams of protein a day, that's only 900 calories. That'll allow even those on a restrictive diet to get plenty of the other macronutrients.

Chances are, in the beginning at least, you'll have to keep track of your protein intake to make sure it's sufficient. A lean, 180 pound man would have to eat *at least* 5 meals with 36 grams of protein in each. Like many "protein" bars and shakes, a sugar-loaded Odwalla "Super Protein" drink with only 13 grams of protein is just not going to cut it. You've got to start reading labels, and doing the simple math.

The key here is to throw out the junk you eat and replace it with quality sources of low-fat protein like skinless chicken and other lean meats like turkey (and even some pork and ground meat), all seafood (canned tuna being the cheapest and easiest), egg whites, all sorts of low fat cold cuts, soy, tofu, some veggie burgers, low fat cheese and other dairy products. Again, just check the labels in your grocery store. You'd be surprised at how many foods are high in protein and low in fat.

Hooya!

WATER

Too often water is an afterthought, and yet no nutrient is more vital or necessary in as great amounts. Maintaining proper hydration is an essential part of healthy living. Every day, we lose 2 - 3 quarts of water through urination, sweating, and breathing.

In addition to helping you build muscle, drinking water can help you fight fat, fever, asthma, arthritis, depression, constipation, bad complexion, stomach aches, or even a stuffy nose. The truth is that you'd be hard pressed to find a malady that isn't eased by imbibing more water.

A man's body is approximately 60% water, and a woman's is about 50%. Consider the fact that you can survive for weeks without food, but only about six days without water. When the water in your body is reduced by just 1%, you get thirsty. At 5%, muscle strength and endurance deteriorate, and you become hot and tired. When the loss reaches 10%, delirium and blurred vision take over. At 20%, you're dead.

Sufficient water intake not only burns calories, but allows your liver to be more efficient at mobilizing and eliminating fat from your body. Water helps to eliminate toxins from the body, and to transport other nutrients into our cells. It is required for a proper balance of vitamins, minerals, and electrolytes, which ensure that your muscles have a full range of motion, prevent muscle spasms and cramping, and regulate the pattern of your heartbeat. By maintaining proper blood density, water helps manage blood pressure, and the movements of fats so they are not deposited as plaque in the blood vessels. Water also wards off food cravings caused by dehydration and thirst.

Never let thirst be your guide. That's like coasting onto an interstate emergency lane with a completely empty gas tank being your indication to put some gasoline in your car. It's already too late. By the time you're actually thirsty, you're already dehydrated.

The commonly accepted rule for water consumption is 1 cup of water 8 times per day, or about 2 quarts or liters a day. Try to carry a water bottle with you whenever you can.

Lastly, as it turns out, standards in the United States regulating bottled water are no more stringent than those for tap water. The best choice, both for you and the environment, is to filter your tap water.

RESTING METABOLIC RATE (RMR)

RMR is the amount of calories needed to sustain all of your body's functions while at rest. RMR accounts for approximately 65% of your body's total calorie consumption, activity burning the remainder. It is governed by several factors. Some are genetically predetermined, while others we can control.

The main factor is lean body mass, which accounts for approximately 80% of our RMR. And there's only one way to affect lean body mass: Build muscle. Our RMR decreases by about 5% every decade after thirty, mainly because of the loss of muscle mass associated with aging. Fortunately, our lean body mass can be controlled through proper nutrition and strength training. It only takes a few months of training to recover one or two decades of decrease in our RMR. Metabolically, muscle is very expensive tissue, even when it is at rest. No matter your age, just two extra pounds of muscle will cause approximately the same amount of calories to be burned—throughout the day, even while at complete rest—as a 45-minute aerobics class.

Another way to positively influence our RMR is to provide our body with a steady flow of nutrients. The body is extremely resourceful, and during times of starvation it adapts by slowing down its RMR. It tries to save every calorie consumed by storing some as fat. Any of the common diets that severely restrict your caloric intake neglect this principal, and that is why people on those diets almost always gain at least their original weight back. When the body receives a regular flow of calories, in the form of frequent meals, it allows the RMR to remain high, and burn those very same calories off.

Frequent meals also utilize the thermal effect of food. Eating temporarily cranks up your metabolism. The more meals you eat in a day, the more consistently your metabolism is boosted. You experience an increase in your RMR for about 5 hours every time you eat. This accounts for 5 - 10% of your total calorie expenditure. Over the long haul this can make quite a difference.

Intense exercise also boosts the metabolism for up to 48 hours after completion. This is one of the main reasons why high-intensity interval training is so much more effective than cardio or steady state training—neither of which is intense enough to have a lasting impact on your RMR.

CALCULATING DAILY CALORIE EXPENDITURE

If you don't feel like making these calculations yourself, on MarkLauren.com you can find an RMR calculator.

To convert your weight in pounds into kilograms (kg) divide your weight in pounds by 2.2. Pounds / 2.2 = kg

To convert height in inches to height in centimeters (cm) multiply your height in inches by 2.54. Inches x 2.54 = cm

Men's RMR

10 x weight (kg) + 6.25 x height (cm) - 5 x age + 5

Women's RMR

10 x weight (kg) + 6.25 x height (cm) - 5 x age - 161

Once you have the caloric output of your RMR, multiply it by one of the following factors that best suit your activity level. The result is your daily calorie expenditure. Anyone following my program exclusively should choose 1.55 (moderately active) as the multiplier.

1.2 = sedentary (little or no exercise)
1.375 = lightly active (light exercise/sports 1-3 days/week)
1.55 = moderately active (moderate exercise/sports 3-5 days/week)
1.725 = very active (hard exercise/sports 6-7 days a week)
1.9 = extra active (very hard exercise/sports and physical job)

---*Hooya!*---

THE FAT AND THE FURIOUS

Try to remember, you're not a hot rod. You don't ever need to "fill 'er up." The difference between feeling "satisfied" and feeling "full" after a meal is about 1,000 calories. Then, even worse, there are about 2,500 calories between feeling full and feeling "stuffed"! So if you go to town on that all-you-can-eat Chinese buffet, and leave the place feeling stuffed, you may have wolfed down as many as 4,000 unneeded calories. A typical reaction is to do some cardio the next day to "burn off those calories." But to burn that many calories with cardio would require, for example, jogging nonstop for 27 hours. The problem is not burning calories, which is done even while you sleep, but that we cram too many calories into our mouth.

Get into the habit of eating until you are no longer hungry, not until you are completely stuffed. Remember, if you follow my advice, you'll be eating again in 2.5 - 3.5 hours. Take your time, chew your food, and relax. It takes 15 - 20 minutes for the body to register how full it actually is. Eating fast and furious can be a hard habit to break. But you'll very quickly notice improved energy and well-being once you make the change to frequent, smaller meals.

LOSING WEIGHT

The bottom line for fat loss: 1) Build some calorie burning muscle through strength training; 2) Create a modest calorie deficit through dietary restraint. As you know, this means eating properly balanced meals and fewer calories than you expend.

As you may not know, every pound of bodyweight contains 3500 calories. So if you want to loose a pound a week, you'd only have to consume 500 calories less than you expend every day (7 x 500 = 3500).

This is done by controlling your calorie intake and burning calories through exercise, day-to-day activity, and by raising your RMR through added muscle, frequent meals, and the post-workout rise in RMR.

Loosing .5 - 1.5 lbs a week is optimal. If you are very overweight, you should be closer to 1.5 pounds a week (750 calorie daily deficit), and if you only have a few pounds to shed, .5 lbs a week is ideal (250 calorie deficit daily).

Taking your time will prevent muscle loss and maximize your chances of keeping the weight off permanently. Don't give in to the temptation of not eating or doing tons of aerobic exercise—both of which will cause muscle loss, and therefore counteract your goal of long term fat loss. Ideally, you want to build muscle in order to increase your RMR. You must do everything in your power to prevent the loss of muscle while loosing weight. If you try to loose weight too quickly, you will not only prevent muscle growth, you'll cause your body to breakdown its existing muscle for fuel. This is going in the wrong direction. Remember, it isn't simply about weight. It's about body composition—less fat and more muscle.

Key Points for weight loss:

· Loose .5 - 1.5 lbs per week by eating 250 - 750 less calories than you burn daily.

· Eat 5 meals per day, every 2.5 - 3.5 hours.

· Maximize your calorie expenditure by building muscle through consistent, short, intense strength training.

· Eat a diet that gives you 1.5 grams of protein per pound of your ideal bodyweight, and split the remaining calories between mostly unsaturated fats and carbs with a low glycemic index. Stay away from processed sugars; they're everywhere!

· Don't starve yourself and don't overeat.

EATING IN AND OUT

Going hungry to a restaurant or party is a common pitfall that can lead to some major overeating, especially since it's these places where you typically consume the most unhealthy food. Unlike when you prepare your meals yourself, you can't control your food's content when you're out on the town. Even if you try to eat the healthiest thing on the menu, you'd be amazed by the amount of butter and oil they throw on just about everything in the kitchen.

A great secret to not overeating at restaurants and parties is to simply eat a small meal right before you leave home. That way, when you get there, you're focused on having fun, instead of waiting for food to fill your belly. Focus on enjoying yourself, the company you're with, and the party or restaurant—not on dieting or gorging yourself. You order less, save more money, and tend to really enjoy what you eat because you're eating to satisfy your taste buds, not your empty stomach.

So don't sweat it if you go out a couple of times a week to eat. Just try to eat as balanced of a meal as you can comfortably, and don't stuff yourself.

All it takes is a small meal beforehand. Just remember, between traveling to the restaurant, being seated, getting menus, ordering and having your food cooked, chances are you're not going to actually be served food for another hour at the very earliest. So think ahead. Don't ever leave your house hungry. Eat a little beforehand, order less, and have more fun.

GAINING WEIGHT

To gain weight, you need to consume more calories than you expend. Whether the surplus of calories is used to build muscle or fat depends largely on whether or not you place a demand for added strength on your body. How do you create such a demand? By *consistently* engaging in short intense bouts of resistance training that consists of mainly compound movements like any type of Push Up, Pull Up or Squat.

Keep a close eye on your body composition. If you notice yourself packing on more fat than you feel comfortable with, back off the calories a bit. On the other hand, if you're not seeing any changes, bump up your calorie intake.

Keep in mind that if you're trying to build serious muscle mass, it's inevitable you'll pack on a little fat at the same time. Don't worry about it too much. Focus on eating enough and gaining strength. Then, after you've got your muscles, shift your focus to loosing body fat to show them off.

Key points to gain weight:

· Consume 500 - 1000 more calories than you expend daily.
· Maintain a well balanced diet. 1.5 grams of protein per pound of bodyweight with an even split of carbs and mostly unsaturated fats for the remaining calories.
· Eat frequent meals, 5 - 6 per day, every 2.5 - 3.5 hours, with plenty of whole pieces of fruit, raw or steamed vegetables, nuts, seeds, meats, fish, and diary.
· Consistently strength train.

MEAL SUPPLEMENTS

If you feed your body regularly throughout the day, your energy levels will remain stable, you'll avoid hunger, and simultaneously fuel your metabolism. But let's face it, most folks are too busy to go find six healthy meals each day. So prepare them the night before, and stick them in your fridge or freezer, either let them defrost over the next day (like sandwiches) or pop them in the microwave, and you're good to go.

Another great method is to balance three whole-food meals with two or three protein shakes or bars. There's no cooking or cleaning involved. Shakes are preferable, since sports bars tend to contain higher amounts of sugar and other unnecessary additives.

If you're looking to bulk up, use a high calorie, "weight gainer" shake. For those trying to slim down, use a supplement that contains a higher ratio of protein to carbs and add one tablespoon of flax seed oil. Beware that most shake supplements get their carbs from maltodextrin which, while it helps thicken up the shake, also has a very high glycemic index. Don't be fooled by marketing that'll have you believe maltodextrin is good because it's a complex carb. If you do use a shake that has maltodextrin, try adding a tablespoon of flax seed oil to slow its absorption.

An easy way to get a meal when you're on the go is to bring protein powder in a bottle and shake it up with some water when you're ready for it. To keep clumps of powder from forming, shake it up with half the required amount of water before shaking it up again with the full amount of water. If your supplement is still clumping up, try using a different brand. It's been my experience that supplements that blend easily also digest easily.

A typical diet that incorporates a meal supplement could go as follows:

Meal 1: Oatmeal, boiled eggs, and half an avocado.
Meal 2: Post workout: Cytogainer or Met-RX.
Meal 3: Tuna, salad with olive oil and balsamic vinaigrette dressing, banana.
Meal 4: Cytogainer or Met-RX with flax seed oil.
Meal 5: Fish with vegetables.

For those who don't like to eat breakfast, try a shake instead. Your body's been fasting throughout the night, and that first meal is important to jumpstart your metabolism and provide needed nutrients. Don't neglect it.

Hooya!

POST WORKOUT MEAL

It's the most important thing you eat and the exception to the rule. As soon as possible, following your workout you need to consume:

- 30 - 50 grams of a lean complete protein like whey, soy, egg, chicken or fish.
- 30 - 50 grams of carbohydrates with a high glycemic index.

Why lean protein? Because fat slows the absorption of protein and carbs. During a brief window of opportunity after your workout, protein synthesis occurs at the highest rate. This is due to the micro-trauma (broken-down muscle tissue) that occurred during your workout. Complete recovery will be optimized if you provide your muscles with a large supply of amino acids—the key components of protein—within 45 minutes after your training session. A whey protein shake is the best post-workout protein choice because it is so rapidly absorbed, and it has the highest efficiency ratio, or availability to the body, of all proteins.

Why carbs with a high glycemic index? Immediately following your workout is the only time to eat carbs that rapidly absorb into the blood stream as the glucose causes an insulin spike. Insulin helps shuttle protein into the muscles, repairing and building new muscle. It is also an important hormone that regulates the storage, replacement, and use of glucose. During a workout, the body uses stored glucose that is in the blood and muscles as fuel for the activity. If the lost glucose isn't refilled within about 45 minutes after training, your body rapidly goes from an anabolic state (muscle growth and repair) to a catabolic state (cannibalizing of the body's muscle for protein and energy). Since insulin signals the body to replenish and store glycogen, and the release of insulin is best triggered by eating foods with a high glycemic index, it makes sense that eating carbohydrates with a high glycemic index, along with some lean protein, is the best post-workout choice.

An effective and convenient post workout meal is a whey or soy protein supplement, which contains maltodextrin, or simple sugars, as its carb source.

PROTEIN POWDER

Unlike some other books, I'm not going to endorse a brand I represent or own. The truth is most protein powder brands are largely interchangeable, so just find the ones you like. What I will say is be careful of the amount of carbohydrates in a protein powder, oftentimes they're packed with sugar. Unless you're looking to gain weight, total carbohydrates should be less than half the amount of protein. Also, a money-saving secret is that it matters little what *kind* of protein you buy, as long as it's a complete protein, meaning that it has all the essential amino acids. Whey, egg, milk, and soy proteins all fit this bill. It makes little difference if your protein has the latest "whey isolate ion-enhanced" mumbo-jumbo in it. 40 grams of whey isolate will have the same effect on building muscle as 40 grams of whey concentrate or soy.

KEEPING A LOG

There's no doubt about it, with practice, eating right becomes second nature. But if you're just getting started it really helps to keep a log. It'll put your diet into perspective and build awareness of everything you put into your body—both *what* you eat and *how much* you eat. Your plan should, at a minimum, take into consideration the following:

· What are your specific goals? If it's weight loss, then what is your ideal weight loss rate (.5 - 1.5 lbs per week)? What is your ideal weight?

· How many calories do you expend?

· How many calories do you need to consume?

· What is your meal plan (what and when)? How do you make your diet fit as conveniently as possibly into your lifestyle?

· Is your diet balanced? It should contain 1.5 grams of protein per pound of bodyweight with the remaining calories coming from an even split of mostly low glycemic carbs and unsaturated fats.

Eating well is primarily about 2 things: How much of each macronutrient we eat and our overall calorie intake. The simplest way to monitor both is to read the nutrition labels on your food packaging. Pay attention to the calories per serving and proportions of macronutrients. I've already shown you which proteins, fats, and carbohydrates are best. See MarkLauren.com for serving sizes, calorie contents, macronutrients, and glycemic indices of common foods.

It is impossible to overemphasize the importance of proper nutrition. A good understanding and application of these dietary fundamentals is absolutely necessary to reach and sustain your fitness goals. Build awareness of what you put in your body, and apply my basic principals. Then, with enough practice, eventually you'll hardly even have to think about it anymore.

Hooya!

TAKING OUT THE GARBAGE

The best way to avoid eating junk is to simply banish it from your home. You won't be tempted to eat poorly, because there's nothing left to be tempted by. Instead you'll find yourself eating wholesome foods, which is *always* what your body is actually craving, even when your mind is not.

7.

COMMON STRENGTH TRAINING MYTHS

SPOT REDUCTION

Ah, yes, that old belief, constantly reinforced by glam mags every summer, that fat loss can be isolated to a particular area of the body. "Want to lose belly fat? Just do some Sit Ups!"

Well, it doesn't work that way. Not at all.

The reality is that if you have fat on your tummy, doing Sit Ups is *not* going to give you a 6-pack. While doing hundreds of Sit Ups every day will indeed build strong abs, it will do nothing to reduce fat in that area alone.

Fat loss can only be achieved in all areas of your body at once, and it can only be achieved by burning more calories than you ingest, and you burn calories most effectively by building muscle. In fact, working your thighs or shoulders will do as much, probably more, than Sit Ups to make you lose fat on your belly (and everywhere else), since they are bigger muscle groups.

Unless you get rid of enough fat all over your body for your abdominal muscles to show through your skin, building strong abs will only push your belly fat out further.

So how do you loose love handles, flabby glutes, or a soft tummy? Eat well and build muscle through strength training. Then, the rate at which each area looses fat is determined by genetics.

MUSCLE CAN TURN INTO FAT

Fat cells and muscle cells perform completely different and separate functions, and one will never transform into the other. When someone becomes "soft" and overweight after being "hard" and muscular, it is because the calorie output no longer exceeds the calorie intake. Largely, this is due to a decreased metabolic rate from the loss of muscle. The loss of muscle is caused by the lack of necessary stimulus. There is no magical transformation of muscle into fat, just a loss of muscle mass and an increase of body fat.

YOUR MUSCLES WILL GET TOO BIG IF YOU DO STRENGTH TRAINING

I've heard it from women especially, all over the world: "I don't want to get too muscular." Some have seen the initial results of strength training and then shied away in fear of becoming the next Ms. Olympia. First off, in case you didn't already know, male and female professional bodybuilders (and most likely some of the bigger guys at your gym) all use steroids and other illegal substances. The human body—yours included—simply will not accrue that kind of muscle mass without serious drugs.

For men and women, the initial gains in muscularity that are common within the first couple of weeks of strength training are largely due to an increase in circulation within the muscles. Similarly, the jumps in strength are mostly due to the body's neurological adaptation to new movements rather than added muscle mass.

The fear that you will accidentally become more muscular than you intended or that you will start growing uncontrollably is unfounded. For women, consistently gaining a half pound of muscle a month is outstanding progress. For men, a pound and a half is comparable. Keep in mind, this will occur under ideal conditions only. A muscular body is built through consistent dedication to strength training and proper nutrition. It won't happen overnight or accidentally.

This brings us to another myth...

WOMEN SHOULD TRAIN DIFFERENTLY THAN MEN

A common misperception is that women will get bulky from strength training. They won't. Not unless they start popping pills and sticking needles in their buttocks.

There is no reason to train differently based purely on your sex. Both sexes gain and lose muscle and fat the same way. It's true, men and women often have different goals. But surprisingly, these different goals can be achieved with the same program.

Most women aren't looking to develop big chests and arms, but rather to firm and tone their entire body, especially their legs and glutes which tend to be the hardest things to maintain as they age. The ironic thing is that they should do exactly the same thing to achieve these goals as men should do to bulk up. Women too often just take their arms along for the ride when they workout. Remember, men and women's muscles are identical, the only difference being in size. It's virtually impossible that a woman would get bulky, muscular arms from doing upper body exercises. Even most steroid-saturated professional female bodybuilders don't have huge upper bodies. Some women continually fail to understand that if they exercised their upper bodies as much as their lower, their tummies would just be that much flatter, and their glutes that much tighter, because they would be increasing their overall lean muscle mass. Again, building and maintaining muscle, alone, is the most effective way to burn fat and calories.

In contrast, the manly man has been taught to hit the bench press, lat pull down machine, squat rack, and other contraptions of bodybuilding that achieve less functional and less physically attractive results than the full array of bodyweight exercises in my programs.

MORE IS BETTER

For some it's intuitive: They think the more you workout, the more you'll grow, and the longer you workout, the better. Since muscle is the most effective fat burning tool we have, we should train without making compromises to our muscular development due to poor nutrition or overtraining. Remember, your muscles grow while you rest.

Overtraining and poor nutrition are easily the most common pitfalls that beginners and experienced fitness enthusiasts alike fall into. It's not possible to say exactly how much is too much, since many factors such as genetics, diet, sleep, training intensity, frequency, and duration all play a role. It's best to watch for the following signs of overtraining: A halt in progress, chronic fatigue, decreased motivation, frequent injuries, and an increased resting heart rate, which is measured first thing in the morning before getting out of bed.

If overtraining is suspected, adjust one or more of the following: Diet, amount of sleep (you should try for 7 - 8 hours per night), training intensity, duration, and frequency.

YOU CAN RESHAPE A MUSCLE BY DOING ISOLATION EXERCISES

Nope.

Your muscles can only get bigger or smaller. The shape that your muscles take, as they change in size, is determined not by the specific exercises you do, but by genetics.

Keep in mind though, that some muscle groups that we often think of as single muscles, such as the shoulders, thighs, or back, can be changed by emphasizing a certain muscle within that muscle group.

The shoulders, for example, can be given that nice heart shape, when viewed from the side, by making the rear deltoid larger, but the shape that your rear deltoid takes can only be controlled to the degree that you make it bigger or smaller.

Similarly, you can make the "teardrop muscle" in your thighs (the smaller one just above and to the inside of your knees), larger by pointing your toes outward during squatting exercises. On the other hand, you can increase the outside "sweep" of your thighs (which makes gives women great bikini legs) by turning your toes slightly inward during any squatting exercise, and therefore focusing more on your *vastus lateralis*.

YOU NEED HIGH REPS FOR DEFINITION AND LOW REPS FOR MASS

Neither your body nor a particular muscle will become more defined by doing a high amount of repetitions of any exercise as opposed to doing low repetitions. How defined a muscle is will be determined by its size and the amount of fat around it, period.

For definition we need to do what most effectively builds muscle and burns fat. Doing high reps in order to burn extra calories is extremely ineffective, and the muscle built will be limited, and we should always remember our greatest calorie burning ally: You guessed it— muscle.

A consistent variety of high-intensity interval training along with proper nutrition is the way to get defined muscles. If too much size is truly an issue, simply cut back on the calories, because the major factor affecting mass is nutrition. Most adult males could do workouts in the low 2-5 rep range on a 1500 calorie diet for the rest of their days without ever gaining any size.

It's true that low rep workouts, consisting of powerful and explosive movements, will build more size (but *not* less definition) than high rep workouts, because the "fast twitch" muscle fibers required in explosive movements are much larger than "slow twitch" fibers required for more enduring tasks. But really, for mass, wouldn't you want to recruit all possible muscle fibers and not just the fast twitch?

Likewise, for "definition"—that is, losing body fat so the striations in your muscles show more—wouldn't you want to recruit all possible muscle fibers, especially since the number one factor affecting our resting metabolic rate, and thus fat loss, is muscle mass?

The only thing you should alter depending on your goal—whether it's to tone or bulk up—is *nutrition*.

STRENGTH TRAINING MAKES YOU BIG
AND CARDIOVASCULAR TRAINING MAKES YOU LEAN

Again, dietary intake is the major factor that regulates body composition. While prolonged moderate pace exercise such as aerobics will help slightly increase your caloric expenditure, it will do little to build muscle. Without strength training, you are neglecting the best fat burning tool in your arsenal: More muscle! I'm sure you're getting the idea by now... Nothing raises the body's resting metabolic rate more effectively than muscle. A few extra pounds of lean muscle will burn approximately the same amount of calories throughout the day that the average aerobics class will. Added muscle makes you burn more calories even while you sleep.

To gain weight, increase your calorie intake and build muscle through strength training.

To get lean, decrease your calorie intake and increase your resting metabolic rate by building muscle.

YOU CAN'T BUILD MUSCLE AND LOSE FAT AT THE SAME TIME

If you're just beginning this program after a long period without much exercise, with proper nutrition, you'll experience gains in strength while losing fat at the same time. For those more advanced athletes, it's tough, but *not* impossible. With a perfect balance of complex carbs, good fats, and enough protein, your body can achieve these seemingly separate goals.

RESTRICTIVE DIETS

People often starve themselves in order to loose weight. That's a no-go!

The body is very resourceful, and it will slow down its metabolic rate in order to compensate for the lack of calories. It tries to hold onto every calorie you consume, since it is unsure when it will be fed again. Then, once you resume your normal caloric intake, your metabolic rate remains slowed down. This is why people who try restrictive diets usually gain their original weight back and often some more too.

The good news is that if you want to lose weight, you should never be hungry. A well balanced diet consisting of small frequent meals (every 2.5 - 3.5 hours) is the key to long term success.

8.   MOTIVATION

IT BLOWS ME AWAY EVERY TIME I walk into a nice home and meet its proud, overweight, out-of-shape owner. They just don't get it. Your real home is *not* your apartment or your house or your city or even your country, but your *body*. It is the only thing you, your soul and your mind, will always live inside of so long as you walk the earth. It is the single most important physical thing in this world you can take care of.

We have a choice: To take care of ourselves, or to simply let time make us worse. And it is right now, at this moment, not later, that we must make this decision. Most people in this world choose to lose. They drag themselves through a second-rate life, overweight and under-energetic. They just let time take its toll. Their waistline increases and their height decreases as they get older and their backs hurt and hunch. Eventually their mobility becomes limited. And they meet their maker well before they should.

Then there are the others, the minority who decide to really, truly do something about their health. They exercise, and they watch what they eat, not obsessively, only just enough. They have an understanding of nutritional basics, and workout about 20 - 30 minutes a day, 4 - 5 times a week—less than 1.2 % of their time—because that is all they will ever need. They meet life's obstacles with physical, mental, and spiritual strength. They care about how they look, and they look good. They thrive on the energy exercise gives them every day. How it washes away so many of the bad things in life—depression, anxiety, nervousness, tension, boredom, impatience... It lets them think easily and clearly. They know how much worse their lives would be if they did not exercise, so they simply don't let that happen. They are in control, not their excuses.

EXCUSES, EXCUSES...

Just look around you at the gym (if you still use a gym, that is). The people who are in the best shape are usually not in an aerobics or yoga class, or being toted from machine to machine by some trainer with a clipboard. They're the ones working out *alone*. The ones who have the drive and knowledge to customize their own strength training routines. Yet even they haven't taken the final step of independence: Walking out of that fitness center and never returning.

So much of what people have learned about fitness only hinders their potential. Fitness centers, classes, trainers, bench presses, dumbbells, machines, and gadgets are all crutches, excuses not to buckle down and reach your optimum level of fitness. The ironic thing is that people often feel they have to put themselves through far harsher and lengthy routines in the gym than the more effective bodyweight programs explained in this book.

I've visited hundreds of gyms in my career. And the proof is in the pudding. I look at the people there. Then I look at my SpecOps troops. The difference is night and day. And you can achieve this difference with an amazingly small sacrifice of your time. I mean, who cannot really find the time or willpower to workout for 20 – 30 minutes, four or five times a week, and completely change their life?

Keep in mind, you can certainly do my program with a buddy, but don't ever depend on a workout partner—that's just another crutch, another excuse not to workout effectively when you're by yourself, whenever you want, wherever you want. 99% of the truly fit men and women I know are the ones who do it by themselves.

You need to build full independence into your regime to be successful over the long term. Only *you* know what you need and when you need it, only *you* feel your muscles, lungs, bones and ligaments. In the end only you can get you into shape. And that's *all* you need: You.

There will never be the "perfect" time and condition to do a workout. You have to create it, just as we all create excuses, every day, every hour, every minute, not to workout.

If you train in the morning, it's the snooze button that rears its ugly head and threatens you with an out-of-shape, second-rate life. When it's time to get up to train or hit snooze, we're faced with a decision. Sleep for an extra thirty minutes or workout. You want to get into the best shape of your life, but you're so tired and you had a long night and today will be even busier and... It goes on. We've all been there.

You want to be in great shape but you also don't want to let go of your comfort for thirty minutes. You want to be leaner but you don't want to go through the hassle of breaking old eating habits. You want to workout but you also want to sit on the couch and relax. The examples are endless. Your mind can be simply awesome at manufacturing excuses. The bottom line is what is more important to you: Your goals or whatever is in the way of you achieving them?

The next time you skip a workout because of some excuse, you'll know why. That excuse was more important to you than the goal you set for yourself. You failed.

I've seen it time and again: Quitting and failing quickly become a habit. It gets easier as we give in to it, while our commitment and resolve are strengthened every time we don't give in to weak-mindedness.

YOU ARE YOUR OWN GYM

The fact is that one of my short workouts pays enormous dividends once it's over: Stress is washed away, your mind and body are revitalized, your self-esteem is lifted, and those feel-good endorphins explode through your body. This is the outcome of letting the world and its excuses wait, and taking a few minutes for yourself. It pays off in spades.

Never giving up and keeping an achiever's attitude is a matter of having a vision. Once you have a clear idea of what you want—whether it's bigger muscles, a thinner waist, better legs, or to do five straight Handstand Push Ups—it's time to plan your work and work your plan.

Failing to plan with the end in mind is a common mistake. In the military, mission planning is done with a "backwards planning" timeline. You start with actions at the objective and plan backwards from that point after thoroughly establishing what the objective is, what criteria must be met for mission success, and how they will be achieved. Then, execution is simply a matter of not giving up.

You already have in your hands an effective training program and sound nutritional advice, a simple tool to get you into the best shape of your life. That is a very real, attainable goal. Consistently training and eating properly will get you there. It really is that easy. The only thing stopping you is you.

Remember, this is not about long workout programs, or some crazy restrictive diet. The minutes spent exercising four or five times a week will be more than made up for with the new efficiency with which you conduct the rest of your life.

There are hundreds of benefits to regularly following an effective physical training program, but one that is often overlooked is your improved ability to serve others. It will not only make you strong and lean, but it will strengthen your resolve. Your friends, loved ones, and coworkers will get a stronger version of you. Take the time to serve yourself, so that you can better serve others. That, above all, is beautiful.

But let's face it, the # 1 reason people want to workout is to look better. You don't see before and after pictures of people's hearts and lungs, or their improved aerobic capacity, or their renewed vigor in their relationships and business. We're all a bit vain and want to look good. So use your vanity to your benefit. Look in the mirror and use that dissatisfaction or pride that you feel to motivate you. As you continue to train you'll see the results: New lines, a new shape, the curves of growing muscles, a hardness you didn't have before. Your body will change. With consistency, you'll start to look better and you will always continue to.

I saw it in Combat Control and Pararescue trainees all the time. The classes would start with what seemed to be boys and by the end there was something different about them. They were muscular, lean, balanced, all around athletes, but there was more. They carried themselves differently. They knew themselves better. They dealt with the enemy within on a daily basis and they were winning because they were still there. Day in and day out, for months they were tried and tested, but they never quit. Those young men valued their performance more than they valued their comfort, and they knew when to ignore the mind's reasoning. They had became their own masters. It showed in everything they did. As it will with you.

You will have command over a stronger, healthier body. Each day you decide what form your body will take through commitment, perseverance, and vision. The dozens of excuses that your mind fabricates when you're tired or short on time are ignored. You press on because you have set a goal, and falling short of your goals is as habit forming as everything else you do in life. You realize that giving in to your excuses becomes easier the more you allow it, and that your resolve strengthens each time you don't. You must temporarily set aside your comfort and train, because you have made a decision to become a better person, one short workout at a time, and that is simply more important than any fatigue or stress that you might be dealing with. It's a small, immediate sacrifice for a long and healthy life.

Hooya!

GET YOUR FOOT IN THE DOOR AND YOUR HANDS ON THE FLOOR

As with many things, the hardest part is often just getting started. Next time you don't feel like training, try tricking yourself. Tell yourself that you're just going to do a few sets of something or a quick 10-minute workout. What you'll find is that usually, after you get warmed-up, you start feeling better, your energy surges, and those few sets turn into a full-blown workout. Worst case, you end up with an abbreviated workout. It's still better than doing nothing!

Heck, if you're really not feeling it, just play around with some exercises. It doesn't always have to be so structured or serious. The great thing is that you don't even have to leave the room you're in. Just drop down and do some Dive Bombers, or lie under your desk and crank out some Let Me Ups, or grab your door and start some Door Pull Ups. I often have workouts where all I do is play around with different exercises. Have fun with it.

Crunched for time? I've done workouts that consisted of 100 non-stop 8-Count Body-builders or Burpees or a mix of the two in a hotel room. The whole workout only lasts about 8 minutes. It's a kick in the butt, but it proves you don't need much time to get a good workout, just a little bit of motivation.

You probably won't get there if you don't know where "there" is.

So what exactly are your goals? And what are the excuses that get in your way?

It's good to write down both your goals and your excuses. Identifying your excuses will make you more aware of them. It'll take the wind out of their sails. It'll make it easier for you to identify those "reasons" for not training for what they really are: Useless excuses that stop you from reaching your goals.

When you write out your goals, make them specific and quantifiable. The more specific the better.

Your overall goal may be just to get fitter, but that's like going to target practice with a blindfold on. Only with more specific, quantifiable goals will you start aiming at real targets. Each goal you set gives you a bull's-eye to aim for. Learning to direct your limited energy toward specific tasks will not only improve your quality of work, it will also increase the likelihood of you achieving what you set out for.

Make sure your goals are realistic. Remember, the tortoise wins the race. It's not about going gung ho for 10 weeks, loosing 15 pounds, and then falling back into your old routine. This book is a tool that will help you make long-term changes for lasting results. If you're trying to cut 20 pounds before your friend's wedding in three weeks, you got the wrong book. (Not to mention that's impossible unless you're losing mostly water weight.)

Also, watch out for conflicting goals, such as stacking on big muscle while trying to drop down ten pant sizes. Those are two opposite directions for your body. Don't get me wrong, you can do both—particularly if you are exercising for the first time in a long time—but each detracts from the other. It's like trying to increase your one rep max on the squat while decreasing your 10 km run time. Each would have better results if done exclusively. The body only has a limited amount of recuperative energy. You do not have separate energy reserves for different tasks. If you're trying to get leaner and gain significant muscle mass, it's best to first train with your emphasis on gaining, and then, only after reaching your desired muscularity, switch to loosing fat.

Your goals should answer at least these two questions:

How much of something do you want to gain, loose, or do?

What is your timeline?

Example:

<u>Goal</u>:

    I want to be fitter. (Too general!)

<u>Better Goals</u>:

    Loose .5 lbs of body fat per week.

    Be able to do all the exercises in the Basic program by my birthday.

    Go one week without chugging pancake syrup.

    Go one whole 10-week program without missing a workout.

<u>Excuses</u>:

    I don't have time.

    I'm too tired.

    I'm in a bad mood.

    I don't feel like it.

    I need to relax.

    I'll start over next week.

    I'll make up for it.

    Bullshit.

After you've written your excuses out, just take a look at them. Remember them and decide now that when you hear these thoughts again, you're going to workout despite them. Know thy enemy! He will take many forms and shapes and have many sneaky spin-offs.

9. INTENSITY

ONE OF THE MOST CRUCIAL, yet commonly neglected aspects of any training regimen is intensity—how hard you're pushing yourself.

My workouts may be short, but some are intense. They require grit and determination. To see the greatest benefits of my proven training method you're going to have to let go of your comfort occasionally. That's the deal. In return, you will look and feel better than ever before.

All those infomercials, with celebs and models smiling their pearly whites while rocking back and forth on some ridiculous contraption, are lying to you. Getting in great shape requires some sacrifices. Not sacrifices of time, but instead putting your goals before your comfort.

There is a huge difference between going through the motions and really putting effort into a workout. I saw it constantly training Special Operations troops. My response to trainees that were not putting out 100%: "You obviously value your comfort more than your performance. Start over!" This would continue until they either gave it their all or quit the program. Unfortunately, we can't all be so blessed as to have a screaming military instructor keeping us motivated (*heh, heh...*), so it's up to you to be mindful of the human tendency toward comfort and not let that stifle your progress.

Whatever you do in life reinforces patterns and habits. Quitting or coasting, when it's time to drive on, reinforces that behavior and makes it more likely that you'll do it again the next time. Likewise, every time you push through discomfort and put your goals before your comfort, your resolve is strengthened. Your behavior *now* directly affects your behavior in the future.

If you find yourself walking away from a workout with a little bit of guilt, telling yourself you could have done better, just resolve to get a few more reps or sets the next time around. Focus on progressing, and know that often, especially the more advanced you are, the difference between making progress and staying in a rut is in those last couple of reps that take every bit of will power to accomplish. Arnold Schwarzenegger once stated that it was the last couple of reps of each set that caused muscle growth. It's here that the elite are separated from the majority.

For many of my exercises I'll give you ways to *kick it up a notch* and move on to a harder variation of an exercise. Of course, there's other ways to increase the resistance as well, as I've already described: Increase or decrease the amount of leverage; perform an exercise on an unstable platform; use pauses at the beginning, end, and/or middle of a movement; turn an exercise into a single limb movement. Using one limb rather than two not only causes more fibers to fire in the targeted muscle, but also works your stabilizing muscles more.

Don't get me wrong, not every workout needs to be a kick in the ass, but without a doubt, there are times when a swift kick is exactly what we need. But not to worry, if you follow my program, you'll be eased into it. It's important to first become proficient at these new movements and develop a fitness base (during which time you'll also make good gains) before you can safely and effectively push your limits during high-intensity workouts. Your body will adapt quickly to these new movements, and there is a great sense of discovery, accomplishment and joy you can look forward to as your mind and body conquer new movements. "Ladders," for example, don't require much intensity and it's actually discouraged that you push yourself to the point of muscular failure, since these workouts are designed to develop movement proficiency and a solid foundation for more intense training. Others, such as Stappers and Tabatas, are meant to be high-intensity.

So how do you know how hard to push yourself for the different workouts that you'll find in this book, and how will you adjust the intensity to suit your abilities? Each of the workouts in this book will be marked with an appropriate intensity rating on a scale from 1 - 4. If you find that any of the sample movements in a program don't allow you to stay within these parameters then feel free to change the actual exercises. Whether a movement is too easy or too difficult matters not. If a particular exercise is getting too easy, and it allows you to exceed the rep scheme for a particular workout, then change to a more challenging variation or exercise.

TAKING IT TO THE LIMIT

In order to build muscle we need to apply the right stimulus, and occasionally it's necessary to take yourself to muscular failure and even beyond, especially the more advanced we become. We just need to be sure to use these techniques very sparingly, since their overuse will quickly lead to overtraining. After taking a set to complete or near failure you can try the following:

- Switch to an easier variation of the same exercise or another exercise that works the same muscles and take that movement to failure. For example, if you're doing Push Ups with your feet on a desk, after you hit muscle failure, try dropping your feet to the floor and once again going until you can't anymore. Or if you're doing them standing on the floor with your hands on a desk, try doing a few more reps with your hands on something higher like a windowsill.

- Try prolonging the last negative movement, a technique I often use. For example, you've just done your last set of Chinese Push Ups to muscle failure, now try lowering your head to the ground as slowly as possible, fighting it the whole way. If you need to, you can also try "cheating" your way back to the fully extended position of the exercise. For example, by dropping your knees to the ground in order to push yourself back up. And then do one super slow negative after "cheating." See if you can make it last 30 seconds!

- Do several more reps using 3 - 5 second negatives, "cheating" your way to the fully extended position of that exercise.

- Hold the fully extended or contracted position as long as you can.

- Intentionally pause for 3 seconds at the most difficult part of a movement. A great way to overcome "sticking points" and develop strength. This is typically halfway through a rep. For example, try pausing with your elbows—forearms and upper arms—at a 90-degreee angle during a set of Push Ups or Pull Ups.

- After muscle failure, crank out a couple of half reps to finish yourself off.

- A combination of any of the above mentioned techniques!

NO PAIN NO GAIN?

Yes, but we have to learn to differentiate between good pain and bad pain. Discomfort caused by muscle fatigue or lactic acid build-up—that burning sensation as your muscles swell and you're giving it your all—is good. It means you're pushing yourself sufficiently hard. Similarly, some muscle soreness the day after a workout means your muscles are recuperating and growing. But discomfort in your joints, bones, tendons, or ligaments, or sharp shooting sensations is bad, and you should stop immediately.

Pushing through that sort of discomfort hurts your fitness, and may force you to take off more time than necessary. Give yourself time to recover from injuries. While recovering, perform exercises that don't aggravate the injury. A common pitfall is continuing to train on a minor injury—instead of taking a couple of days off to heal—then next thing you know it becomes a chronic injury that puts you down for weeks or months. Never train through "bad" pain.

There's a fine line between hard and dumb. Don't push until minor injuries become major ones, but at the same time, don't let minor injuries get in the way of you reaching your fitness goals. It's easy to let the old "I'm injured" excuse keep you from training when it shouldn't. Instead, train around a minor injury, being sure not to do anything that aggravates it. For instance, if your right elbow is bothering you, simply use movements that do not stress it.

I have a link to an excellent source of information about causes, symptoms, and treatments for a wide variety of sports injuries at <u>MarkLauren.com</u>. Of course, nothing can or should replace the expert eye of a qualified professional. Remember, when in doubt, always seek the advice of your health professional.

10.   TRAINING TOOLS

ONCE YOU LEARN THE EXERCISES and get a real feel for them you'll no doubt want to construct your own programs that can be changed and modified in seemingly infinite ways. You're not in the gym, there's no one to impress. Don't train your ego. Train your muscles to perform the exercises correctly.

Sets and repetitions (reps) are the most common method of structuring workouts. A **repetition** is one complete movement of a particular exercise. Doing nine Push Ups translates to nine reps.

A **set** is one complete series of reps from beginning to end. The completion of nine Push Ups is one set of nine reps.

When deciphering a workout routine, the number of sets are written first and the number of reps second. 3 x 12 is three sets of twelve reps each.

Reaching **failure** means that the set is to be done until another rep is not humanly possible. It requires a lot of intensity, drive, and determination, but it is well worth the effort. It is that very last rep that sends the message to your body that there is a demand for greater strength and more muscle. All other sets and reps are for the purpose of bringing you to that final point of failure, and other than that, the only use they have are to warm you up, improve technique, and raise your heart rate.

Each muscle group only needs to be worked once a week. While the program splits them into four sections: Push, Pull, Core, and Legs, you can also replicate a standard gym training regimen. Break your muscles up into:

- Shoulders (8 to 12 sets)
- Triceps (6 to 9 sets)
- Chest (8 to 12 sets)
- Lats (8 to 12 sets)
- Biceps and forearms (6 to 9 sets)
- Core (6 to 9 sets)
- Thighs (8 to 12 sets)
- Calves (8 to 12 sets)

If you tackle two muscle groups a day, you're only working out 4 days a week. Sometimes I like to spend less time per day, but more days overall, really cranking up the intensity of the sole muscle group I work that day. I might workout 5 or even 7 times a week, but only do one body part each day.

You can do the standard, tried and true, typical strength training program: Do a set to failure, rest for 2 - 3 minutes, then another set, doing 3 or 4 sets each of 3 or 4 different exercises for each muscle group.

But for those who want to throw some spice into your regimen, here are some of my favorite training techniques. Have fun with these, use them to construct your own programs, and any and all can be combined with methods found under *Taking It to the Limit* in the last section.

Ladders: Perform one rep of any exercise, rest, perform two reps, rest, perform three reps... Keep increasing your reps until going any higher would cause you to hit muscle failure on subsequent sets. Once you've reached that point, come back down without repeating the highest number. The rest intervals are the time it just took you to perform your reps. So you'll have more rest as the numbers get higher, and less rest as the numbers get lower on the way back down to one.

Try doing them for ten minutes with a single exercise. If you've reached the bottom of your Ladder (1 rep) and the set time hasn't expired, simply start another ladder.

It's a great, high-volume, low-intensity method to build movement proficiency of any exercise. Train yourself to perform the exercises correctly. If you reach muscle failure at any point during your ladder workout, you went too high before coming back down. It's okay to perform a ladder workout in the low rep range—possibly even using repeated single reps towards the end of the workout, in order to avoid hitting failure. Exercises where you alternate sides are done by performing the designated number of reps on both sides before resting.

Push-Pull Ladder: Perform a pushing movement immediately following a pulling movement using the Ladder format, without rest between sets. Using Pull Ups and Push Ups is a favorite in the Combat Control community.

Stappers: Choose any number of exercises and repetitions, and repeat as many cycles as possible in 20 minutes. Usually three or four different exercises is best. Be sure to keep your reps low enough not to hit failure during the first couple of rounds of sets. It's okay to take short breaks because of muscle failure, but try to keep rest to a minimum. This one can be a real butt kicker.

Supersets: Perform one exercise immediately after another. This is best done with different exercises that emphasize the same muscle group. For example, doing a set of Let Me

Ins after a set of Door Pull Ups is a fantastic way to stimulate all the muscle fibers of your back, biceps and forearms.

Interval Sets: Usually done with 1, 2, or 3-minute intervals. Begin the exercise as soon as the interval starts, go until failure, and then rest until the interval is elapsed, at which point you begin the next set.

The Easy Gleason: With a continuously running clock do 1 Pull Up the first minute, 2 Pull Ups the second minute, 3 Pull Ups the third minute... continuing as long as you are able. You can do this with any exercise.

Timed Sets: Do as many repetitions as possible of one exercise in a given amount of time. For example, how many Dive Bombers can you do in 10 minutes, no matter how many sets it takes you? Or do 20 second sets, followed by 40 seconds of rest, every minute for 20 minutes. By increasing or decreasing the duration of sets, timed sets can effectively be used to develop power and/or muscular endurance. The shorter the set is, the higher the intensity should be and vice-versa. It can be likened to a 50-yard sprint compared to a 3-mile run. Short sets build power; longer sets build muscular endurance.

Timed Workout: The opposite: Perform any given workout as quickly as possible. For example, see how quickly you can do 50 Dive Bombers, regardless of how many sets it takes.

Tabatas: 20 seconds of exercise followed by 10 seconds of rest, for 8 rounds, for a total of 4 minutes. You should do as many reps as possible in each 20 second set. If failure is reached during a 20-second work period, just pause at the bottom or top of the movement until the 20 seconds is up. This high intensity training is superb in a time crunch. If you want a great workout, select just three different exercises that work the same muscle group, and do three Tabatas with a couple of minutes of rest in between. That's only 15 minutes total workout time and you're done!

52 Pick-Up: Shuffle a deck of cards. Ace through 4 are Push exercises, 5 through 7 are Pull, 8 though 10 Core, face cards are Legs. Overturn one card at a time, do a set of *any* of the appropriate exercises in your ability group, then turn over the next card. Go through the whole deck, taking as little time between sets as possible.

Circuit Training: Perform a series of exercises, usually with relatively short rest intervals between sets and exercises. Work all major muscle groups and perform at least 2 sets per group. This allows a large number of sets, reps, and exercises to be done in a short amount of time for those with limited time or patience. An effective way of organizing a circuit workout is to designate work and rest intervals to a series of exercises and sets. 45 on/30 off, for example, means that all sets are performed for 45 seconds with 30 second rest periods. The exercises, duration, and intensity of the sets will determine whether it is a workout focused on power, muscular endurance, or both.

Active Recovery: Simply perform any variety of back-to-back exercises with low to moderate-intensity and little or no rest between sets. The idea here is to maintain your target heart range for 20 – 60 minutes.

An easy formula to calculate maximum target heart range is to subtract your age from 170. Minimum target heart range is 10 less than this. For example, with a 30-year old:

170 – 30 = 140, 140 – 10 = 130; Target Heart Range = 130 to 140 beats per minute.

Creativity: Don't be afraid to combine any of the above mentioned techniques in as many variations as you can create.

Got some favorites I missed? Or even some you invented yourself? Shoot me an email at MarkLauren.com, and I'll name them after you.

11.   THE EXERCISES

HERE IT IS: THE BIBLE OF BODYWEIGHT EXERCISES. The essence of the book.

Many of these 111 exercises I developed and named myself, others are little known gems, and still others are classics modified in new ways. Each exercise description details a single repetition. Obviously, you should do multiple repetitions for multiple sets with rest in between sets. For more advanced athletes, typically each set should be done until you hit muscle failure and cannot do another rep.

You can find "Variations" at the end of many exercises to make them easier, as well as ways to "Kick it up a notch." As you can accomplish more and more reps, switch to a harder variation of the same exercise, and then eventually switch to a more difficult exercise altogether.

Please remember that each exercise is not simply about pushing or pulling yourself up as hard and fast as possible. Slow, controlled, negative movements are just as important in developing muscle.

Breathing properly is also crucial for optimal performance and safety. In general, you want to exhale as your muscles contract, and inhale as your muscles stretch. Take Push Ups, for example: As you lower yourself down (muscles stretching) you should inhale, and as you push up (muscles contracting), exhale. Simple. A different method of breathing should be used when doing power movements that require maximum exertion, like weighted Pistols, incline One-Arm or Planche Push Ups, or Spidermans. For that, see MarkLauren.com.

The exercises are split into four sections: PUSH, PULL, CORE, and LEGS & GLUTES. If you work out four days a week, it's a good idea to devote one day exclusively to each of these. Also, at the end, I've laid out some great all-around "Butt Kickers," movements that develop most muscles in your body.

Below the name of the exercise, you'll find the muscle groups that each exercise develops, in a descending order of emphasis. But keep in mind many of these exercises actually work much more than just these muscles. Unlike using machines and dumbbells, which tend to only work one muscle group, bodyweight exercises tie your muscles together in a functional way by incorporating many at once, including your stabilizer muscles, leaving nothing lacking and nothing out of proportion. For example, unlike the bench press, Push Ups work much more than just your chest, shoulders and triceps. In fact, some of my trainees have stopped doing core exercises altogether, and instead just do my Push Up variations. And believe me when I tell you these guys and gals have 6-packs.

We also labeled each exercise with a number from 1 to 4, indicating the level of fitness required, 1 being an easier movement, 4 a far more difficult one. This is not to say that an elite athlete cannot benefit greatly from using exercises that have a rating of 1, just that they will need to do more repetitions, or make them more difficult in one of the previously mentioned ways. Also, many exercises have variable ratings, depending on which variation you choose. These numbers are merely a suggestion, a guide. No one should ever think themselves only a "1" or a "3" and therefore only try exercises with those numbers.

I encourage anyone to pick and choose from this encyclopedia and construct your own fitness program, or incorporate these exercises into your existing regimen. If you already have a good workout program in the gym, you can find exercises here that mirror your gym exercises, ones that work the same muscles (and more), and then simply substitute them for your usual gym exercises (and cancel your membership!).

If you don't have a routine yet, or want to try something new—or if you would like to follow a simple, specific program rather than mining through so many exercises—I encourage you to embark on one of my fitness programs, which I detail after the exercises. Workout just 4 - 5 times a week for 20 - 30 minutes, for 10-week cycles. There's four programs for four different fitness levels, each utilizing the science of "periodization" to keep your body progressing, preventing burning out or getting stuck in a rut.

---*Hooya!*---

THE PARTS ARE GREATER THAN THE WHOLE

Doing exercises a single limb at a time is one of the most effective ways to build all the components of fitness. Not only does it correct any imbalance which goes unnoticed when both limbs are working at the same time, but one limb working alone has more than half the power of both limbs moving together. This is because when you work both limbs at the same time a defense mechanism (called the *bilateral deficit*) kicks in, hampering some of your motor units in an effort to prevent injury to your body during your heaviest lifts. Thus unilateral movements like One-Legged Squats or One-Handed Let Me Ins, are safer and superior to doing a similar movement with two limbs using more reps or harder leverage.

Index of Exercises

PUSH Exercises

Most PUSH exercises focus primarily on your pectorals, shoulders, and triceps. But one of the many great things about doing them with only your bodyweight is that they work so many more muscles as well. For example, unlike bench pressing, doing Push Ups will strengthen your abs and the rest of your core. In fact, once you progress to the more intense types of Push Ups, like Semi-Planche or One-Arm Push Ups, you won't need to work your core separately at all.

Unlike the other three sections, we'll lead this PUSH chapter with an exercise you already know—the Classic Push Up. You'll notice the Push Up description is long, but this is not your daddy's Push Up. And once you understand the many variations, particularly altering your leverage, you'll see that there's almost countless ways to do a Push Up. For those who don't think they can ever do a single good Push Up, I'll show you how to easily work into it. The more advanced fitness enthusiast can move on to exercises like Dive Bombers, which incorporate the Sun Salutation yoga posture, and I'll walk you through Handstand and One-Arm Push Ups, and even insane strength tests like the Planche Push Up. I round these off with a few workouts that focus squarely on your pecs, then we'll move on to triceps, and finally shoulders and traps.

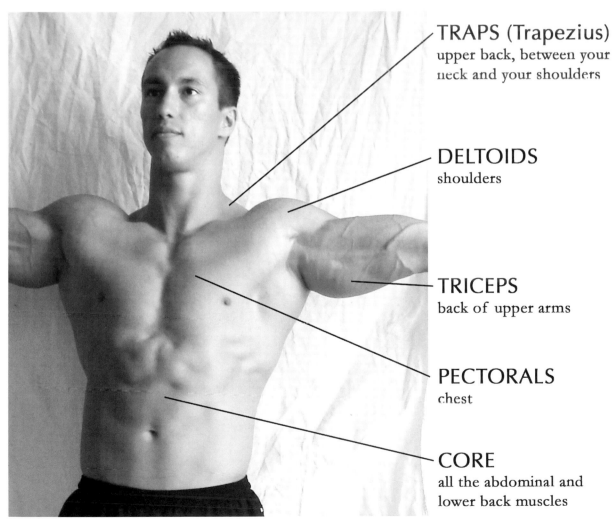

TRAPS (Trapezius)
upper back, between your
neck and your shoulders

DELTOIDS
shoulders

TRICEPS
back of upper arms

PECTORALS
chest

CORE
all the abdominal and
lower back muscles

Rocking Chairs

pectorals, triceps, deltoids, core (1)

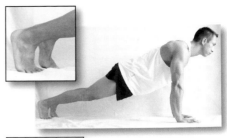

Start in the beginning position of a Classic Push Up, your body in a perfect line, your arms straight and your hands directly beneath your shoulders upon the floor. Now push your body slowly forward six to ten inches with your toes, keeping your arms straight. Return slowly back to the starting position.

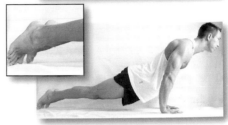

Ready to kick it up a notch? Again, start in the beginning position of a Classic Push Up, but lower your body to within five inches of the floor, as though you're indeed doing a Push Up. Once you're in the bottom position, move your body forward, parallel to the floor, six to ten inches with your toes. See how long you can do this for. Or you can complete a Push Up after each rep.

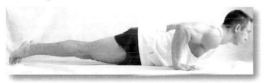

Bear Walk

shoulders, pectorals, triceps, traps, core (1)

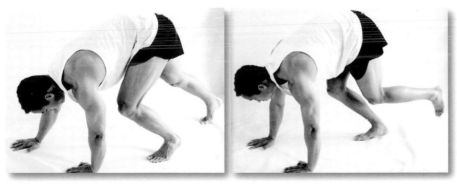

Simply place your hands on the ground a few feet in front of your toes, and start crawling on your hands and feet. Have some fun. This is a good exercise for a beginner, because it uses so many muscles at once. You'll start to feel it after a while. It's also a great exercise to do at the end of a PUSH workout, to really finish off your entire upper body.

PUSH UPS

Any exercise where you are using your arms to push yourself or an object against gravity will strengthen not only your pectorals, but your shoulders and triceps as well.

With any type of Push Up, putting your hands closer together than shoulder-width will put more emphasis on your triceps. To really concentrate on your triceps, form a triangle with your fingers (index fingers touching each other and thumbs touching each other), and keep your elbows in close to your ribs throughout the movement.

Similarly, a wider than shoulder-width hand position focuses more on your pecs.

Putting your feet on a surface will make any Push Up more difficult and put more emphasis on your shoulders. The higher the surface, the harder it gets, and the more you'll be shifting the concentration to your shoulders.

Keep in mind that each pectoral is one muscle. Despite what you might hear in the gym or read in magazine articles about certain exercises that work the inside or outside, upper or lower pectorals, it is physiologically impossible to stimulate growth in any part of the pectoral muscle without doing so in the whole muscle. Thus, Deep Push Ups will not develop your outer pectorals more than the inner portions. Similarly, putting your feet up on something when you do Push Ups (much like doing an incline bench press in the gym) will not put any more focus on the upper regions of your pectorals than it will the lower regions. But elevating your feet *will* put added emphasis on your front deltoids, which the pectorals overlap, and thus added shoulder development may push out the upper pectoral region.

Most of you are probably familiar with the Classic Push Up. The following explanation is for those new to the exercise, those who have difficulty with it, and those who may need to work on their form, whether they know it or not. As with all exercises, you will only reap their maximum strength and muscle benefits with perfect form. Just remember, you're not in the gym anymore, there's no one to impress by throwing heavy plates around, and in the process weakening or injuring yourself.

Classic Push Ups

pectorals, triceps, deltoids, core (1-4)

Lie down on your stomach, feet together, with your hands directly below your shoulders. Push yourself up off the ground. Throughout the entire movement, your body should be in a straight line. From your heels to your neck, nothing should be bent. Be especially certain not to let your pelvis drop toward the ground, or let your butt stick up in the air at all. Weak form means a weak core. Keep your midsection tight! Let your chest fall until your upper arms are at least parallel to the floor. A perfect Push Up is done by touching your chest to the ground.

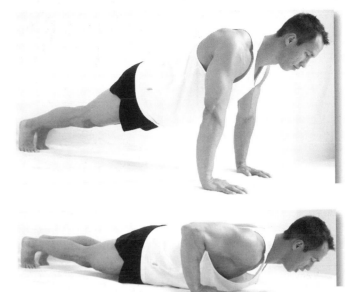

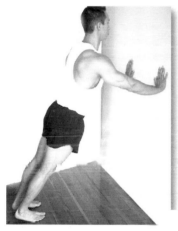

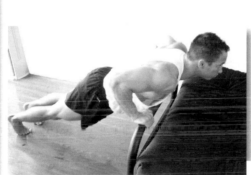

Variations: If you're not ready for the Classic Push Up, you can start working up to it by placing your hands on an elevated surface, like a table, bureau, armrest of a futon or couch, or a wall. The higher the surface, the easier it gets. This is a superior method of working up to a Classic Push Up than simply putting your knees on the ground and doing Push Ups, because it will help you develop the important core strength needed.

Similarly, putting your feet up makes it more difficult, as well as focusing more attention on your shoulders. From a telephone book to a coffee table to your bed, the higher it is, the harder it gets.

A great way to further strengthen your lower back (lumbar region), is to only have one leg touching a surface, and to hold your other leg up in the air while you do Push Ups. You can alternate legs between reps or sets.

Ready to kick it up a notch? Put your feet up on any unstable platform, such as a basketball. This will help strengthen your core as well as recruit more stabilizer muscles in you arms.

Wherever your feet are, you can always increase the resistance further by putting some extra weight on your back like a book-filled backpack, your son, girlfriend or wife, whatever you can think up.

Wide Grip Push Ups

pectorals, shoulders, triceps, core (2-3)

Just like a Classic Push Up, except you place your hands farther apart than shoulder-width, thus shifting the emphasis to your pectorals.

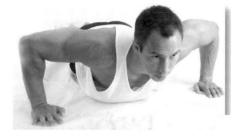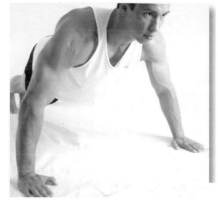

Shoulder Drop Push Ups

pectorals, triceps, deltoids, core (2-3)

A great way to hit all your PUSH muscles from new angles. This exercise is just like a Classic Push Up, except that you bring one shoulder down to the ground, while keeping the other as high as possible. Do one side to failure, then the other immediately after. On the next set, switch the starting side.

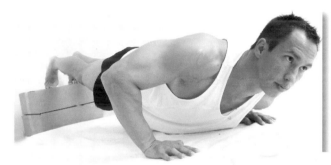

Deep Push Ups

pectorals, triceps, deltoids, core (2-3)

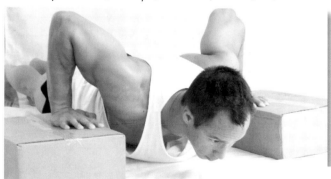

Find two even surfaces to place your hands on: phone books, reams of paper, foot stools, full boxes, whatever. Or you can use three similar chairs, one for your feet, and one for each hand so that you can drop your chest down as far as possible between them in the bottom portion of the movement, really stretching your pectorals and deltoids. Do a Classic Push Up, but bring your chest down until it is fully stretched. Again, keep your body locked in a straight line the whole time.

Variation: Putting your feet up on a surface like a low table or bed makes a big difference here.

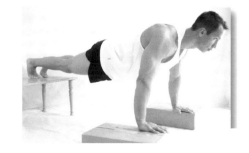

Staggered Hands Push Ups

pectorals, shoulders, triceps, core (1-3)

This is performed just like a Classic Push Up except one hand is slightly forward of the normal position and the other hand is slightly back. Switch hand positions every other set. This is a great exercise for attacking your muscles with varying stimulus.

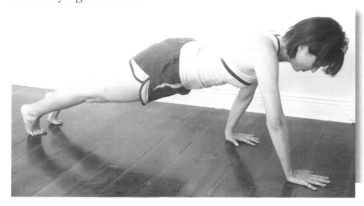

Variations: Elevate your feet or hands to make this exercise harder or easier.

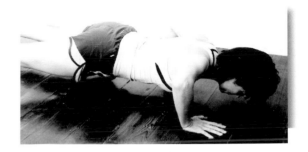

Shove Offs

pectorals, shoulders, triceps (1-4)

Great for developing power! Stand in front of an elevated surface, such as a sturdy desk, mantle, or windowsill. Then fall forward catching yourself on the surface with your hands, palms down. Lower yourself in a controlled manner until the surface is touching your lower chest. Push yourself up as quickly as possible, pushing off the surface with enough force to bring yourself back up to the standing position without ever bending at the waist.

Variation: The lower the surface is, the harder the shove needs to be, and the more power you'll build.

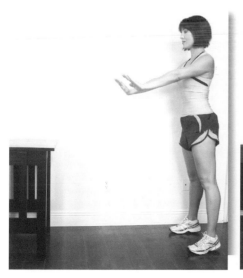
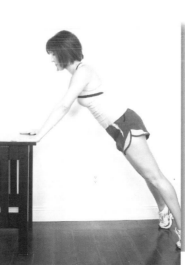
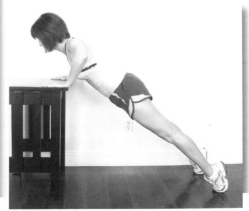

Bouncing Push Ups

pectorals, triceps, deltoids, core (3)

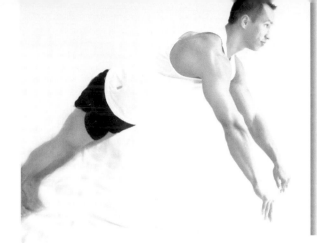

This exercise builds explosive power. Same as a Classic Push Up, but push yourself up so hard and fast that your hands come up off the ground at the top of the movement when your arms are straight. When you return to Earth, don't let your hands crash back down on the floor. Instead, land with your fingertips, then palms, then let your arms bend as your body falls back down in a controlled manner, until it's time to explode back up again.

Ready to kick it up a notch: Try doing these up onto phone books placed just outside or inside of your hands, and then pushing off the books and landing with your hands back down on the ground, alternating back and forth between the floor and the books.

Mountain Climbers

shoulders, abs, core stability (2)

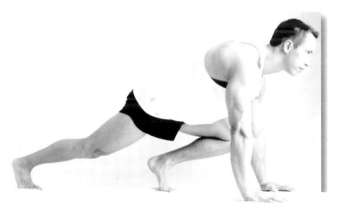

Start in the Classic Push Up position, keeping your neck, spine, tailbone, and legs all in a straight line, and your elbows straight with your arms locked out and hands directly below your shoulders. Keeping the rest of your body totally locked in place, bring your left knee into your chest and place it on the ground.

Straighten your left leg again and "jump" it to the starting position while, *at the same time,* pulling your right leg up toward your chest. Repeat this at a fast pace for a set time or number of reps. It should be as though you are running in place while in the Push Up position.

Basketball Push Ups (3)

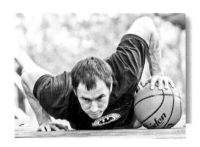

This will put extra emphasis on your stabilizer muscles and core. This exercise is the same as a Classic Push Up, except you balance one hand on a basketball. Bring the shoulder of the arm that is not holding the basketball as close to the ground as possible. The shoulder of the arm that is holding the basketball will only come down to the basketball. For each set you do, switch which arm holds the basketball.

Ready to kick it up a notch? Try putting both hands on one ball to emphasize the triceps or roll the basketball from hand to hand after each rep. You can also put both hands on different basketballs and come down until your chest is fully stretched.

Pec Crawl

deltoids, core, pectorals, triceps (3)

It's best to have a smooth, hard floor for this one. Either wear thick, soft socks, or put a folded towel beneath your toes. If you don't have access to a smooth floor, you can do this on a carpet, but you'll need to wear sneakers.

Start in the Classic Push Up position and crawl forward, using only your arms, dragging yourself on the balls of your feet. (If you're doing this on a carpet, point your toes straight back so that your shoe soles are facing the ceiling and drag yourself on the tops of your feet.) You may bend your elbows, but never beyond 90 degrees. Keep going until muscle failure. If you only have a small room to work in, just quickly turn back around every time you hit the wall.

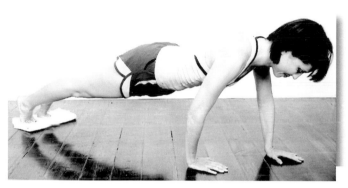 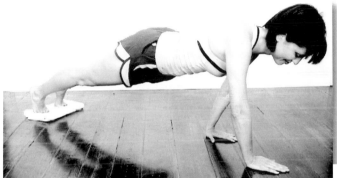

Half Dive Bomber

shoulders, triceps, pectorals, traps (3-4)

Start like you would normally for a Dive Bomber, with your butt in the air, hands on the ground about three or four feet in front of your toes, and your arms locked out and in line with your back. Lower your shoulders, then swoop your chest to the ground, stopping once your chest is between your hands, and from there, return to the starting position. It's like doing a bodyweight "Arnold Press," only using more muscles.

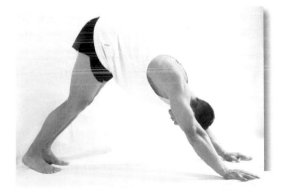

Ready to kick it up a notch? Moving your legs closer to your hands will make this one more difficult. Try it with your hands just five hand lengths in front of your feet. Naturally, the more you move your legs closer to your hands, the more your butt will remain in the air at the bottom portion of the movement. Do them on your fists to increase your range of motion. Put a folded towel beneath your fists for comfort.

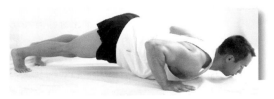

Dive Bombers

pectorals, triceps, deltoids, core (3-4)

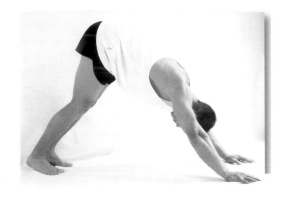

This modified "Indian Push Up" incorporates the *Surya Namaskar* (or "Sun Salutation") yoga posture. It will blast your chest, triceps and shoulders like nothing you would find in a gym, as well as increase your spine flexibility and strengthen your core.

With your legs straight and feet spread a few inches apart, bend over at the waist and put your hands on the ground, about three to four feet in front of your toes as you would for Classic Push Ups. But instead of beginning with your body in a straight line above the ground like a Classic Push Up, push your butt as far as possible into the air, keeping your arms straight and in a line with your back.

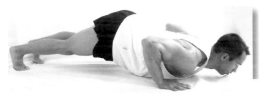

Sticking your chest out, swoop your upper body down in an arc so that your chest almost brushes the floor (at which point you should be in the bottom position of a Classic Push Up), then sweep your head and shoulders up as high as possible, until your back is fully arched and you're staring straight ahead, with your pelvis only a couple inches off the ground.

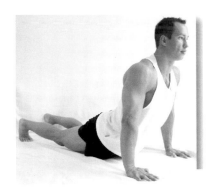

Reverse the motion, again sweeping your chest close to the ground (so that you are again in the bottom position of a Classic Push Up), and only then pushing your body back—this is the hardest part—until your arms are straight and in line with your back and your butt's up in the air again. Maintaining an inverse arch in your back throughout the movement will help elongate your spine and stretch your hamstrings and calves.

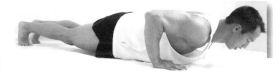

Variation: To make it easier, try spreading your feet wider than shoulder-width apart. To make it a lot easier, do them with your hands on a raised surface like a coffee table.

Also, from the bottom position, with your back arched and your chest and eyes facing forward, you can simply lift your butt back in the air without properly reversing the entire motion, if that portion of the movement is too difficult or you're getting tired. This is a bit like raising dumbbells straight out in front of you—only it requires more muscles—great for your front deltoids. Knocking out ten of these is a great way to finish off a set of proper Dive Bombers after you've reached failure.

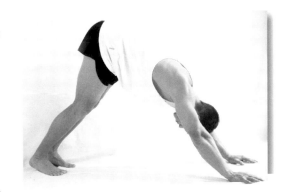

Ready to kick it up a notch? Do Dive Bombers with only one leg on the ground.

Semi-Planche Push Up

the entire upper body with special focus on the chest, shoulders, triceps and core (4)

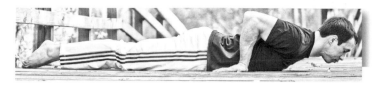

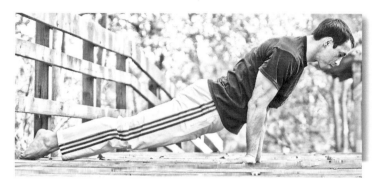

Make sure you're properly warmed-up before doing this exercise.

Lie flat on your stomach, your toes pointed on the ground, and place your hands, palms down, near your waist so that your fingers are pointing back toward your toes. Push yourself up until your arms are straight. Only your hands and the tips of your toes should be touching the ground. The key here is to lean forward as much as possible, bending slightly at the waist but keeping your back straight. Your toes will slide forward a couple inches as you execute this movement so you may want to wear socks or shoes to protect your feet. Then lower your torso back to the ground in a controlled manner.

Variations This exercise gets easier if you start with your hands further forward than waist level, closer to your ribs.

Ready to kick it up a notch? Put your feet up on a low surface like a phone book. Increase the height of the surface as you get stronger.

You should also try keeping only one leg on the ground, the other in the air. Lean forward and put as little weight as possible on the leg that's on the ground As you get better and better at these Push Ups you'll eventually be able to lift your foot off the floor, and you'll be ready for the ultimate Push Up: The Planche.

Planche Push Up (4)

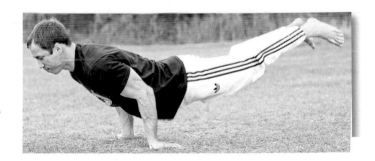

Works everything in your body from your traps down to your glutes with emphasis on the chest, shoulders, and core. This is it—the ultimate Push Up.

As with Semi-Planche Push Ups, you should always be thoroughly warmed-up. Lie flat on your stomach, your toes pointed on the ground, and place your hands with palms down near your waist so that your fingers are pointing back toward your toes. Keeping your body straight, push yourself entirely off the ground until your arms are nearly straight. Nothing should be touching the ground but your hands. Lower yourself back to the ground in a controlled manner.

One-Arm Push Ups

works almost everything, especially your shoulders, triceps, pecs, abs, obliques and lower back (4)

One of the greatest exercises on earth. But unfortunately this is not one you can just muscle your way into. It is not simply a natural progression from mastering other types of Push Ups. I've seen plenty of guys that could knock out 80 perfect non-stop Push Ups, and yet they didn't have the strength and coordination to do a single proper One-Arm Push Up. So don't be disappointed if you can't do one right now. I'll show you how you to work into it.

First you always want to warm up a bit by cranking out an easy set of regular Push Ups. It's best to start practicing One-Arm Push Ups with your feet on the floor and your hand on an elevated surface like a chair, table, desk, bureau, or window sill. Then, as you get stronger, place your hands on progressively lower surfaces, until they're on the floor.

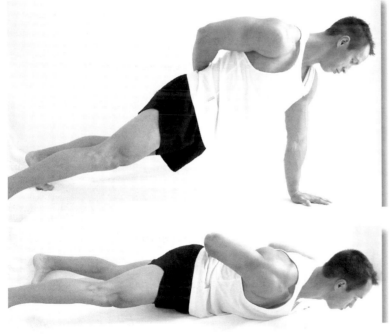

Lean over and place your hands on the surface in front of you as if you're going to do a Classic Push Up on it, only spread your feet a little wider than shoulder-width apart, and put your hands closer together than shoulder-width. Then take one hand and place it behind your back. Spread the fingers of your working hand wide to help balance. Always keeping your shoulders parallel to the ground, come down as far as possible before pushing yourself back up.

You need to keep the elbow of your working arm tucked into your ribs. Focus your weight on the outside edge of your palm, below your pinky finger. And pay special attention to keeping your shoulders squared and down away from your neck. You should remain squarely on your toes throughout the movement.

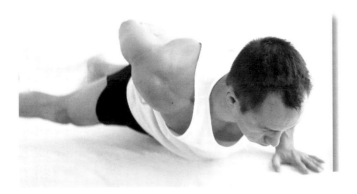

It has an unusual feel to it because of the strong twisting force placed on the midsection. That is what makes this movement so spectacular, and why it will strengthen your abs and lower back so much. The key here is to keep your midsection as rigid as possible. Your natural tendency will be for your body to twist—don't let it! Your body can no longer be only the sum of its parts. It must be one whole—every muscle tightly knit into its surrounding muscles. Flex every part of your body. Your entire body must be rigid, from fingertips to toes. It even helps to make a tight fist with your non-working hand behind your back.

To make your core strong and prevent injury, just before beginning the first repetition, inhale to about half capacity and hold it. Then flex your butt cheeks and your abs, slightly tucking your pubic bone in. This engages your lower back muscles and protects your spine.

Keep practicing until you can come all the way down until your chest almost touches the surface. Once you can do five good reps with each arm, find a lower surface to practice on.

As with other new and difficult compound movements the key to success is lots and lots of frequent, light practice. Try to do 10 to 15 sets spread over the day, each day, but only do about half the reps you need to hit failure. Keep it easy. You're training your body to perfect the form, rather than trying to blast your muscles (for now). Once you've got the form down, you can start getting real workouts, going to failure as you would with any exercise.

Ready to kick it up a notch? To increase the difficulty and focus more on your shoulders, elevate your feet. Or try lifting the same leg of the arm that is on the floor. You can also try doing One-Arm Dive Bombers!

Pec Flies

pectorals, core, shoulders (4)

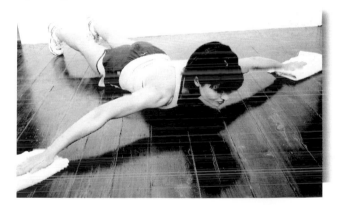

You'll need a smooth, hard floor and two small towels, folded to fit the size of your hands.

Start out lying on your belly, your legs straight, toes up on the floor facing forward, and your arms straight out to either side of you, so that your body is in a cross with your palms down, and a towel folded under each hand.

Keeping your arms as straight as possible, slide your hands together. Your body should remain rigid, and not bend at the waist at all, as you come up off the ground.

Slowly, in a controlled manner, slide your hands apart until your chest just barely touches the floor. Try to bend your elbows as little as possible throughout the movement.

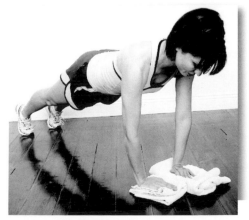

TRICEPS

Your Triceps make up 2/3 of your upper arm, with your biceps making up the remainder. So whether you're a guy looking to fill your shirt sleeves with muscles, a girl seeking to avoid getting flabby upper arms, or anyone in between, we've got just the stuff for you.

Seated Dips

triceps (1-3)

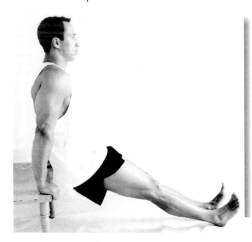

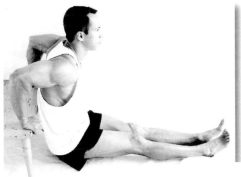

Find a horizontal surface between knee and waist-level. The lower the surface is, the more difficult this exercise gets, but it can't be below knee level. A table, chair, futon or couch armrest will all do the trick. With your back to the surface, place your palms on the edge of the surface behind you, your knuckles pointing forward. Walk your legs forward until they are straight out in front of you and your butt is only a couple inches from the surface.

Lower your body straight down bending only at the elbows and shoulders, until your upper arms are parallel to the floor, really stretching your triceps. Your forearms should stay perpendicular to the floor. Your back should stay only a couple inches out from the surface. Push yourself back up until your arms are straight again.

Variation: You can make this easier by bending your knees, bringing your feet closer in and putting them flat on the floor in front of you.

Ready to kick it up a notch? Putting your feet up on a chair, box, bed, table or other surface makes this more difficult. You can also pile some weight on your lap.

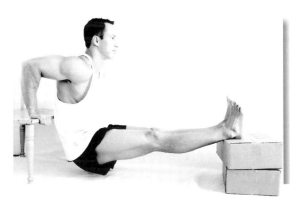

Side Triceps Extensions

triceps, with a minor focus on the obliques (3)

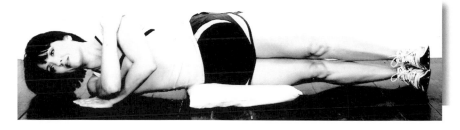

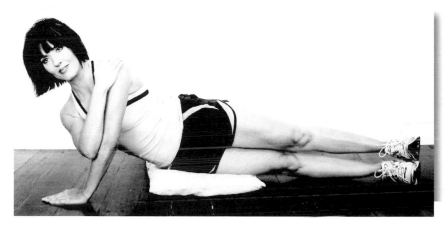

Lie down on your right side so that your body is in a straight line. If you're on a hard floor, put a pillow under your hip for comfort. Take your right hand and grab your left shoulder with it, so that your right arm is bent over your chest. Place your left hand on the ground, fingers pointing toward your head, below your right shoulder. Bending only at the waist, push your upper body up off the ground until your left arm is straight. Lower yourself in a controlled manner back to the starting position. When you're finished with a set, turn over and switch sides.

Crab Walk

works pretty much your whole back side with emphasis on your triceps (1)

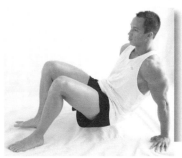

Start by sitting on the floor with your knees bent in front of you. Place both hands, palms down, on the floor at your side and lift your butt off the ground. Now start "crab walking" forward or backwards. Have some fun with this one.

Hip Raiser

triceps, shoulders, glutes and hamstrings (2)

Sit on the ground with your back straight up and your legs straight out. Put your arms to your sides, your palms flat on the ground on either side of your butt.

Keeping your arms straight, raise your pelvis upward so that the soles of your feet now are flat on the floor, until your knees are bent at a 90-degree angle above your feet, and your body—from your shoulders down through your hips and upper thighs—is in a straight line. Let your head fall backwards so that you are looking at the ceiling, and squeeze your glutes. Hold this position for three seconds before slowly returning to the starting position.

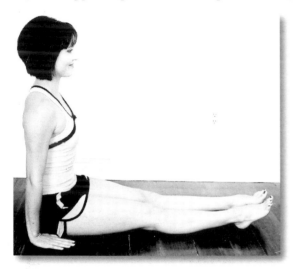

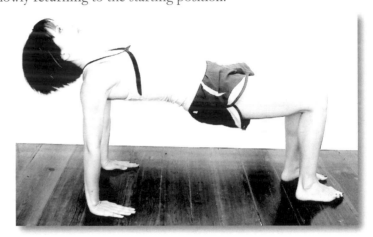

Air Plunges

triceps, lower abs (3-4)

Lie flat on your back with your arms to your side bracing yourself against the ground. Lift your legs straight up until they are perpendicular to the floor. Using your arms to push against the ground, raise your hips off the ground *as high as you can*, keeping your legs pointed up. Lower your hips slowly.

Ready to kick it up a notch? Hold your hips up in the top position for three seconds before lowering them.

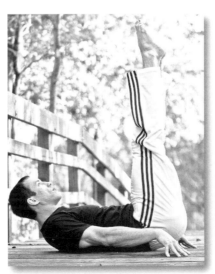

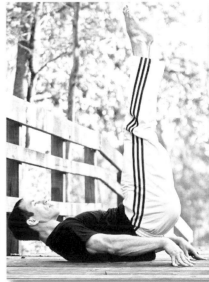

Close Grip Push Ups

triceps, pectorals, shoulders, core (2-4)

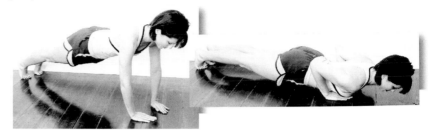

Just like a Classic Push Up, except your hands should be much closer, about one or two hand widths apart. Be sure to keep your elbows in toward your body at the bottom of the movement. The higher you raise your legs the more difficult this becomes. Alternatively, you can put your hands up on an elevated surface to make it easier.

Chinese Push Ups

triceps, deltoids (2-4)

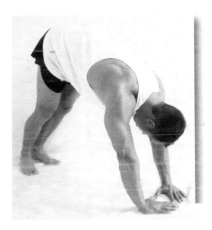

Standing with your heels together, bend over and count five hand lengths away from your feet on the ground in front of you, then form a diamond with your hands there. The tips of your index fingers and thumbs should be touching. Bend at the hips so that you form a 90 degree angle between your torso and your legs. Keeping everything but your arms in a fixed position, your back straight and your butt in the air, bend your arms at the elbow until the top of your head almost touches the ground between your hands. Keep your legs as straight as you comfortably can throughout the movement. Push yourself back up to the starting position.

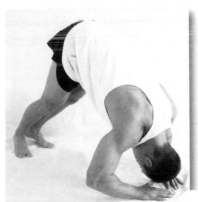

Variation: You can make this exercise easier by placing your hands on an elevated surface. Placing your feet on an elevated surface will this exercise more difficult. Be sure to keep your butt way up in the air and a 90-degree bend in the waist regardless of the variation.

Get In Line

triceps, core, shoulders, pectorals (3-4)

This one is also like a Classic Push Up, but for one very important difference: your hands are in the same vertical line with each other, rather than the same horizontal line. One hand should be under your sternum, the other hand under your forehead. Be sure to keep your elbows in tight to your body throughout the movement, and try to come all the way down until your chest touches your lower hand. Switch your hands half way through your set, or switch every other set.

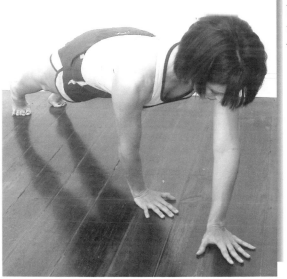
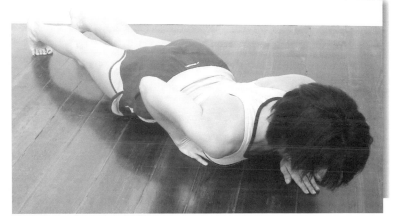

Variation: To make this a bit easier, you can place your hands *almost*, but not quite, in a vertical line. Imagine there is an invisible vertical line on the floor running down the center of your body. Place your hands so that they are on either side of this imaginary vertical line—your right hand just to the right of the imaginary line, left hand to the left. This is a great way to begin doing this exercise until you develop the strength and balance required to align your hands vertically.

Ready to kick it up a notch? If your right hand is the one under your sternum, lift your left leg up in the air, off the ground or surface you're using. Switch legs when you switch hands. Doing these with your feet elevated on a coffee table or something really makes a big difference too.

Surface Triceps Extensions

triceps, core (3-4)

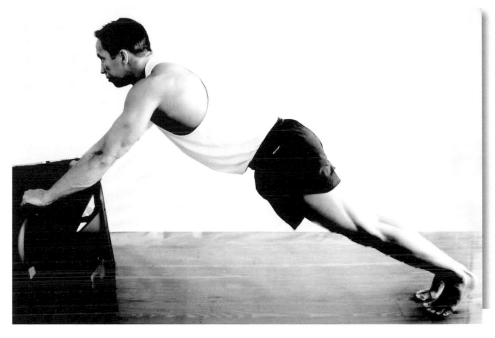

The best exercise for fully stretching and strengthening the triceps.

Find a fixed horizontal surface about waist level, like a stable chair, couch, railing, table, mantle, window sill, or a futon armrest like I use in the pictures. Grasp the surface with an overhand grip, with your hands shoulder-width apart. Lock your arms out to support your weight, then step back a little further than in a Push Up position above the surface.

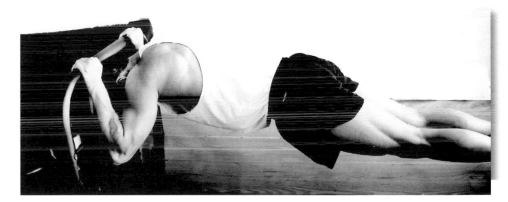

Keeping your body totally straight throughout the movement, bend your arms at the elbow and lower your body until your head comes down just below your hands. Your feet must have been positioned far back enough so that your head clears the surface. When you reach the maximum stretch in your triceps, press forward with your arms and raise yourself back to the starting position with your arms locked straight out.

Be sure to keep your midsection tight in order to prevent bending at the waist. And also be certain to keep your elbows pointed straight down through the movement. Resist the temptation to let them go out to the sides.

Variation: Beginners should try it using something as high as face level, like the top of a bureau or a mantle. The lower the surface is, the more difficult this exercise becomes.

Dips

triceps, pectorals (2-4)

Find any two stable surfaces that are, or can be positioned, a couple of feet apart. The two surfaces should be equal in height (or at least somewhat close) and at least waist high. Kitchen counters, bed posts, high tables, desks, bureaus, bookcases, a window sill, and/or stools can all work.

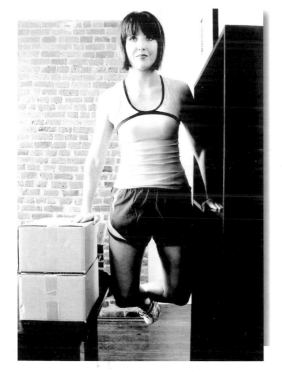

Place a palm on each surface, lock your arms out straight to your sides, bend your knees and suspend your body between the surfaces. Lower yourself as far as possible, your knees suspended in the air above the ground, and then push yourself back up. Again, only your elbows and shoulders should bend. Be sure not to swing your legs.

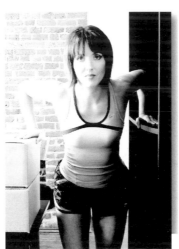

It's okay to use two surfaces that are not quite equal in height. For example, sometimes I do these by putting one hand on my mantle, the other on the back of a chair. Just be sure to switch sides every other set.

Variations: You can push off the ground with your legs lightly to assist yourself and make it easier. Or put a chair behind you, and with knees bent, put your feet on the chair and use it to help push yourself up. If you can, try to pick your legs up off the surface during the negative part of the movement, and control your fall back down. It's a great way to build up to doing these unassisted.

Ready to kick it up a notch? You can wear a weighted backpack to make this exercise harder.

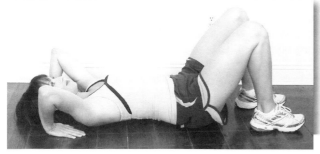

Inverse Push Ups

triceps, traps, deltoids, glutes, lower back (3-4)

Lie down on your back, with your legs bent, knees pointing at the ceiling, and your feet flat on the floor. Place your hands besides your head so that your palms are flat on the floor and your fingers point toward your feet. Your elbows should be pointing out and upwards.

Push your entire body up so that your butt comes off the ground until your arms are almost straight. Arch your back until your shoulders and upper chest are in a line with your arms.

Slowly lower yourself until your back is again touching the floor.

Remember to exhale when you come up off the floor and to inhale when you return to the floor.

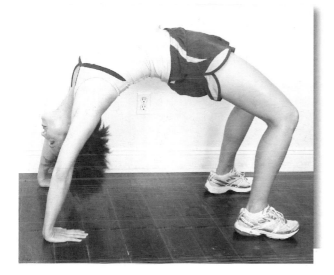

Ready to kick it up a notch? You can transform this movement into a great triceps exercise by holding the peak position, and only lowering your head to the floor, as shown in the photo at right, then pushing yourself up again, for as many reps as you can manage.

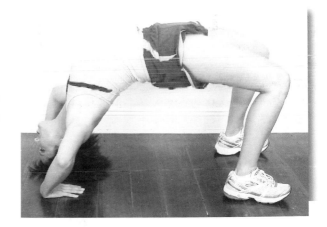

SHOULDERS

The shoulder girdle is primarily made up of the trapezius and three different muscle heads: rear, side, and front deltoids. Only by developing all three heads will you build strong, toned and rounded shoulders

Arm Rotations

shoulders (1)

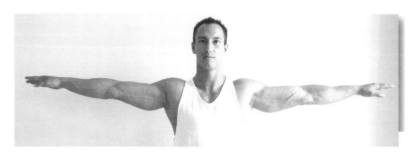

This is a great shoulder warm-up and cool-down, before and after more intense exercises. It's also good for those who are just now getting back into exercise, either after an injury, or in older age. I've gotta admit though, I've conducted more than a few smoke sessions where intolerable numbers of only these have been done to obliterate trainees.

Standing, make small or large circles while holding your arms straight out to both sides of your body. Go forwards for ten rotations, then backwards for ten.

Variations: Making circles with your arms pointed straight in front of you will shift the focus to your front deltoids. And if you bend over, with your arms straight out to either side and flap them up and down the emphasis will be on your rear deltoids. You can also do arm rotations while holding your arms above your head.

Military Press

shoulders, triceps (2-4)

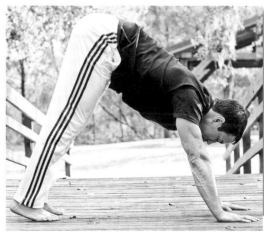

Similar to a Chinese Push Up, except your hands are shoulder-width apart.

Ready to kick it up a notch? Place your hands on a raised surface or surfaces, allowing your head to come below your hands, increasing your range of motion. For example, pull a chair close to a couch or futon armrest, put your hands on the armrest, put your feet up on the chair, bend at the waist so your butt sticks up in the air, legs and back straight, and lower your shoulders until the armrest touches the back of your neck.

You can also put your feet on a chair and your hands on two other chairs, and bring your head and shoulders down between the chairs at the bottom of the movement. Or put a couple of full boxes, dictionaries or phone books on the floor and use those.

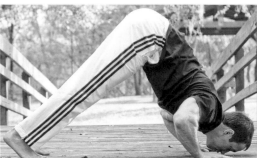

YOU ARE YOUR OWN GYM

The Roof is on Fire

shoulders, triceps, pectorals (3-4)

This one blasts your shoulders, with secondary emphasis on your pecs and triceps. It may seem like a piece of cake... until you actually try it.

Do a single, perfect Push Up.

Get on your knees.

Push your hands straight up into the air four times, as though you're raising an invisible weight from your shoulders.

Do two Push Ups.

Push your hands up into the air *eight* times.

Continue adding one push at a time, and multiplying the amount of Push Ups by four for the amount of hand raises you do in the air after each set. For instance, if you can get up to seven Push Ups, you will follow that with 28 hand raises.

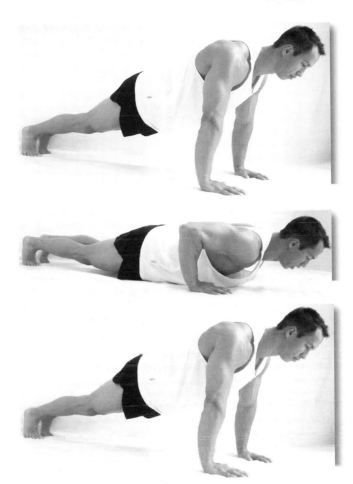

When you can no longer do another Push Up (and your deltoids are burning like hell), pyramid back down to one, again doing four times the amount of hand raises as Push Ups. For instance, if you were able get up to 6 Push Ups, but then barely failed on your seventh, follow that with 28 (7 x 4) hand raises, then go back down to 6 Push Ups, followed by 24 hand raises, then 5 Push Ups, 20 hand raises and so on until you get down to a single Push Up and 4 hand raises and you're done! If you can get up to seven Push Ups this exercise will take about ten minutes total. Remember, the stronger you get the longer it'll take.

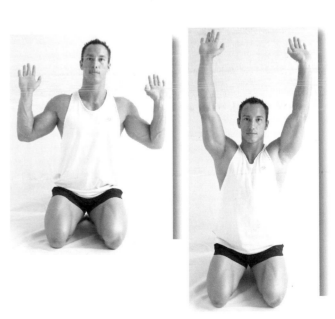

Overhead Press

shoulders, traps, triceps (1-4)

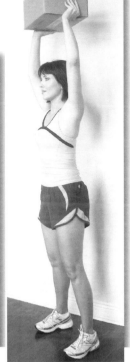
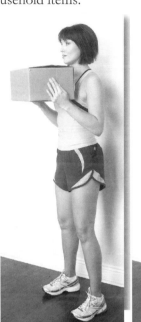

Okay, so this isn't a bodyweight exercise, but it can be easily done with household items.

Standing with feet shoulder-width apart, hold any heavy item, such as a weighted backpack or loaded box, to your chest. You can even use something like a large armchair, holding it upside down by the arms. The more unstable the weight, the more it works your muscles. Using different amounts of weight will obviously change this movement's intensity.

Keep your abs tight and back straight, and press the object straight overhead from your chest until your arms are locked.

At the top of the movement, shrug your shoulders up as high as possible and hold it for a 1 - 2 second contraction.

Lower the object in a controlled manner back to your chest.

Ready to kick it up a notch? Try doing an Overhead Press while at the bottom of a Squat, Front or Back Lunge, or Bulgarian Split Squat.

Thumbs Up

rear deltoids, lower back (2-3)

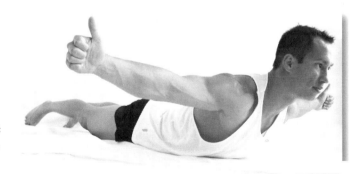

Lying flat on your stomach, put your arms straight out to either side. Make two fists with your thumbs pointed up. Then lift your shoulders and head off the ground and raise your straight arms as high as absolutely possible. Do multiple reps of these, holding your arms at the top of the movement, really squeezing your shoulders, for three seconds each time.

Ready to kick it up a notch? Try simply pushing your arms up for as long as you can, then relax for fifteen seconds and repeat.

Lateral Shoulder Raises

shoulders, with special focus on the side deltoids (1-4)

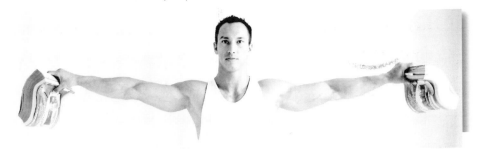

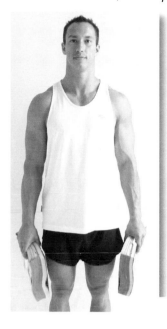

While these are best done holding onto some sort of weight, the important thing is that you need very little weight to really blast your shoulders if your form is perfect. Depending on your strength, holding anything from a couple of soup cans to milk jugs to full grocery bags to filled buckets will do the trick.

Stand with your feet shoulder-width apart and your arms down to your sides. Keeping your elbows straight, palms down, raise both your arms straight out to either side until they are at shoulder height. At the top of the movement, point your thumbs down towards the ground slightly. Hold for two seconds. Then slowly lower your hands back down to your side and repeat.

Variation: To work your traps, extend your range of motion by moving your arms in a full 180-degree arc and touch your hands (or soup cans or water jugs) over your head. As your hands rise above parallel to the floor, twist your hands so that your thumbs are pointing up.

Bent-Over Lateral Raises

shoulders, with special focus on the rear deltoids (1-4)

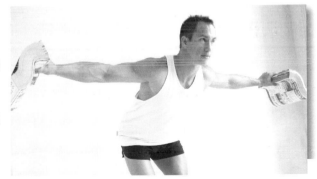

You won't need to hold much weight at all to perform these properly. They're the same as Lateral Shoulder Raises, only bend over at the waist about 45 degrees, keeping your back straight. When doing this exercise, be sure to focus on the contraction at the top of the movement. Imagine that you're squeezing a golf ball between your shoulder blades and hold each contraction for 1-3 seconds. This exercise is great for developing the rear delts, which are a key to good shoulder development. Well-developed shoulders should be heart-shaped from the profile view, yet this is rarely the case, because most people neglect their rear delts, focusing instead only on the side and front delts.

Variation: You can also do these sitting in a chair or on the edge of a couch or bed or other surface. Just be sure to keep your back straight (chest out) and your waist bent at about a 45-degree angle.

Front Shoulder Raises

shoulders, with special focus on the front deltoids (1-4)

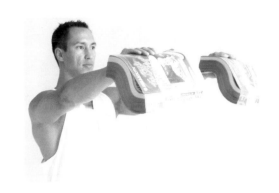

Same as Lateral Shoulder Raises only bring your arms up straight in front of you until they are at face level.

Shrugs and Kisses

traps, side deltoids (1-4)

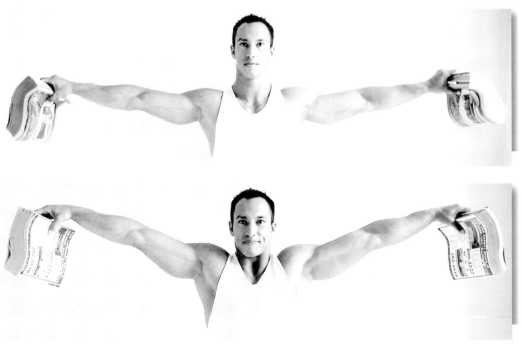

Standing, put your arms straight out to either side (like you're being crucified). Lift only your shoulders up toward your ears, as high as absolutely possible and hold for 5-10 seconds. Really squeeze it! While keeping your arms up, lower your shoulders and repeat.

Ready to kick it up a notch? Hold gallons of milk, water jugs, phone books, soup cans, cinder blocks, backpacks filled with rocks, or anything else.

Handstand Push Ups (4)

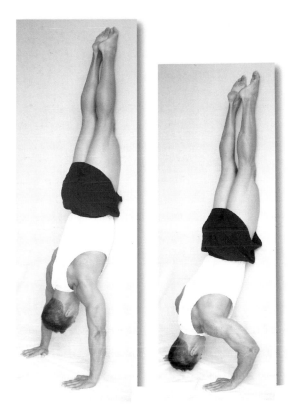

The daddy of them all. While these incorporate virtually every major muscle group in your body, primary focus is on the shoulders, with secondary focus on the triceps and core.

Essentially, you're doing a military shoulder press with your own bodyweight. Unless you can find a wall (such as one outdoors) that can be marked up slightly, you'll want to wear socks or non-marking shoes for this exercise. Bare feet will eventually leave smudges, though they can easily be cleaned off.

With your back to the wall, get down on your hands and knees so that your hands are about 3 feet from the wall and your heels are touching the wall behind you. One leg at a time, put your feet up against the wall behind you, then walk your feet up as high as possible on the wall. Only your hands, with elbows straight, will be touching the ground. Now walk your hands back toward the wall until they are about a foot away from it, letting your legs slide straight up the wall as you bring your body closer to it. You should now be in the perfect handstand position, with your body in a perfectly straight line, from your hands to your feet.

Lower yourself in a slow, controlled motion, until your head almost touches the ground between your hands. Push yourself back up until your elbows are nearly locked. Hold your upper body straight and your core tight as you perform each rep, avoiding the tendency to arch your back.

There are different ways to come out of the handstand. You can keep your butt in the air and simply swing your legs down one at a time to the side, then stand up, almost as if you were doing a cartwheel. Or, if you still have the strength you can walk your hands out away from the wall, and your legs down the wall, simply reversing the method by which you got into the handstand.

If doing regular Handstand Push Ups is a bit much, and you need to get used to the head rush as well, try just holding yourself up in a static handstand against the wall for set periods, like 15 - 30 seconds at a time.

Variation: To focus attention on your triceps, keep your hands close together and form a triangle with your fingers. You can also try doing shrugs while in the handstand position for added trap development.

And once you get good at doing Handstand Push Ups you can try doing static One-Handed Handstands. Place one hand below your head and lift the other hand up off the ground. Maintain this position as long as possible, and then switch to the other hand. Spreading your legs during the exercise is helpful. This really blasts your shoulders and stabilizer muscles.

Ready to Kick it up a Notch? Lower yourself until your nose lightly touches the ground.

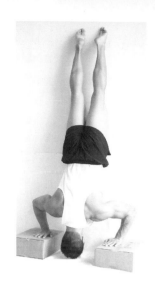

Once you get strong enough, you can increase your range of motion by putting your hands on elevated surfaces like phone books, cinder blocks, or chairs, and bringing your head down in between the surfaces as far as possible. Be sure to use only very stable surfaces.

Try doing Handstand Push Ups facing *away* from the wall. Start out standing, facing the wall. Bend over and place your hands about 6 - 9 inches from the wall with your fingers facing the wall, and then kick your feet up and overhead. Try to maintain control of your legs and don't bang your heels against the wall if you can help it. This method of mounting the wall will prepare you for getting into a handstand without the help of a wall. Execute the movement the same way as a regular Handstand Push Up. In order to get out of this supported handstand position drop one leg at a time in a controlled manner and stand up.

Arms strong as legs…

Handstand Training

Ever wanted to do a handstand? It's a great way to have some fun while blasting your shoulder strength through the stratosphere.

Handstands are one of the best exercises for developing every single muscle in the shoulder girdle. Of course, if you're like most people, doing a handstand doesn't exactly come naturally. So I'm going to show you how. It'll take some real diligence. But your training is not simply a means to an end, because it's exactly this training that will yield the results. Finally doing a freestanding handstand is only the icing on the cake. Your effort and time will be rewarded by well-developed traps, broad shoulders, thick triceps, improved balance, and greater coordination.

Let's walk (on our hands) through the steps…

First you have to master the bodyweight Military Press. See the description for Military Presses above if you need a refresher. Keep your hands shoulder-width apart, with a 90-degree bend at your waist. Remember, the higher your hands are in relation to your feet the easier the exercise will be. If you need to, start out with your feet on the ground and your hands on an elevated surface like a coffee table. As you get stronger, find lower and lower surfaces until eventually your hands are on the ground. Now you're ready to start elevating your feet. Keep practicing, putting your feet up higher and higher as you get stronger, until you're able to walk your feet up a wall and you are in a supported handstand position.

You're halfway there. Now perform Handstand Push Ups while supported against the wall. Then, learn to do them with your back facing the wall. Then practice holding a static handstand there. Try doing three minutes with as little rest and as few breaks as possible. You can use a clock or simply count the seconds—but try to avoid the temptation to count faster and faster as it become more and more difficult. Lastly, once you can do that, hold a static One-Arm Handstand against the wall. Switch arms, back and forth, until you've done three minutes total.

Now you've got the *strength* necessary to hold an unsupported handstand. So it's time to develop the *balance* needed. For most people, this is the biggest hurdle. But it's only a matter of patience and consistency.

First, practice holding a handstand with the wall there to catch you. Place your hands about 6 inches from the wall with your fingers facing the wall, and kick your feet over-head. Try to maintain control of your legs and don't bang your feet against the wall. Now, gently kick your feet away from the wall, and try to hold an unsupported handstand for as long as possible. In the beginning, this may only be a fraction of a second. Keep pushing your heels off the wall, trying to get a real feel for the balance you'll need. At first it will seem impossible. But practice, practice, practice is the secret. Do a lot of easy but frequent handstand training.

Doing a handstand requires a lot of balance and coordination, and light, constant, frequent training will develop these skills better than hard infrequent training. Maybe you've got a particular spot or wall you use to do your handstand training. Well, get into the habit of trying an unsupported handstand every single time you walk by that spot, anywhere from 5 to 20 times a day.

Work on maintaining control of your legs. Keep your legs together and toes pointed straight up. Besides making your handstand look more impressive, keeping your legs from floundering will lead to greater control.

When you get to the point where you can hold an unsupported handstand for a couple of seconds, it's time to take the wall away. Be sure to practice on a carpet, because you're going to fall. You must learn to recover without hurting yourself. That means being able to do a front roll as soon as you lose your balance. To do a front roll bend at the elbows in a controlled manner, tuck your chin into your chest, loosely tuck your legs, and roll forward onto your butt then your legs.

You'll be getting into the handstand position using the same method used to mount the wall when your back is facing it, only there will be no wall there. While practicing your handstands, pay special attention to the position of your legs and head and how they affect your balance. Again, spend some time every day trying to do a handstand without worrying about getting a good workout. Take your time.

Just keep practicing kicking your feet up and trying to hold it over and over and over until you get tired. It's great exercise. Even if you can only get into position and hold it for a second or not at all. Keep doing it. You've got to take some tumbles in order to learn. You try and fall and try and fall and try again. It's how I learned to ride a bike as well. You don't need anyone holding you. You need stubbornness. Consistent training is key. Eventually you'll fall less and less. And then one day, you'll get it. You'll be one in a million—one of the few, elite humans on this earth who can hold an unsupported handstand.

Now all that's left to do is try walking on your hands. And when you can do that, crank out some unsupported Handstand Push Ups—the pinnacle of all shoulder exercises!

PULL Exercises

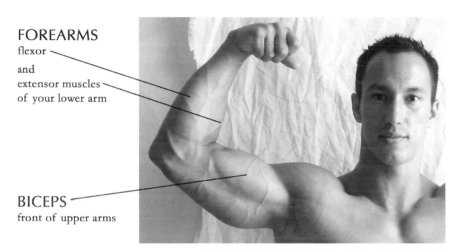

FOREARMS
flexor
and
extensor muscles
of your lower arm

BICEPS
front of upper arms

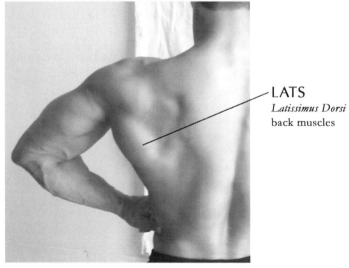

LATS
Latissimus Dorsi
back muscles

PULL exercises emphasize all those upper body muscles that PUSH ones don't. There's fewer separate exercises in this PULL section than other sections, but more variations, including ones that make it possible for virtually anyone to benefit from these exercises—from those just getting into fitness for the first time to gymnasts or bodybuilders. For example, don't worry if you cannot do a perfect Pull Up right now. Under the Variations section I will show you how to work up to this crucial strength builder.

Get to know each of these PULL exercises intimately and you'll see how many different ways there are of doing them—shifting the emphasis between different sides of your forearms, biceps, and portions of your back and even rear deltoids. They're all the exercises you need to build all the strength you want.

Let Me In's

lats, biceps, forearms, rear deltoids (1-4)

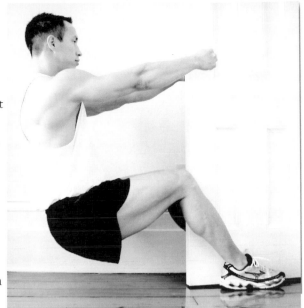

The best overall exercise for your biceps and lats. I'm going to lay out several different ways to do this one, which will shift the focus onto different muscles, as well as modify this exercise's intensity. But first, the basics:

Facing the outer, side edge of an open door, grab hold of the door-knobs on either side of it with each hand.

Place your feet on either side of the door, pressing the door between them. Your heels should be directly below the doorknobs, so that you're straddling the door. You need to be sure to have good traction with the floor, so it helps to wear shoes.

Lean back. Straighten your arms. Bend your knees. Stick your butt out. Create a right angle between your straight spine and your thighs.

Keeping your spine and thighs locked at a 90-degree angle, and your feet flat on the ground (keep those toes down!), pull your chest up until it touches the end of the door. Really squeeze your shoulder blades together. Let yourself back down in a controlled motion, stretching your arms and shoulder blades out as far as possible at the bottom of the movement, always maintaining a 90-degree angle between your thighs and your upper body.

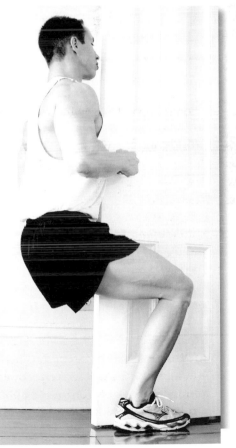

Variations: To make this exercise easier, move your feet back. You can even start with your toes at the door's edge. As you develop more strength, move your feet forward, inch by inch. Keep in mind that the further forward your feet are, in comparison to your hands, the more difficult this exercise becomes.

You can do these over or under-handed, or by using a side grip. Doing them over-handed, palms facing down, places more emphasis on the outsides of your forearms (extensors). Doing them with a side grip, so that your palms are facing in toward the door will place even more emphasis on the outsides of your forearms. While executing these with an under-handed grip will shift the focus to the insides of your forearms (flexors).

Keeping your elbows tucked down and into your ribs, really squeezing your shoulder blades at the top of the movement, and stretching them out wide at the bottom portion, concentrates this exercise more on your back. Pulling your chest into your hands will work the upper back, rear delts and biceps more than pulling your belly into your hands, which shifts the attention to your lower back.

To increase your grip strength, you can hook a towel around the door-knobs, as shown, and grip it close to the door-knobs as possible. Twist your wrists so that your palms turn slightly upward (supination) as you pull yourself in toward the door, thus recruiting different forearm muscles and working your biceps from different angles.

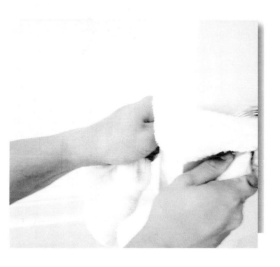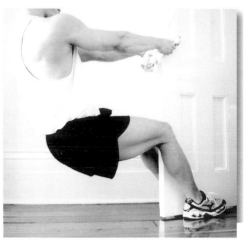

For an easier grip, you can loop a larger towel, or a rope, around the door knobs and tie the ends together, creating a small loop to hold onto.

To increase the resistance, if you wrap a normal-sized towel around the door knobs and grip it a full foot away from the door knobs, while keeping your feet directly below the door knobs, it makes it more difficult and really blasts your biceps and back. Again, the further forward your feet are in relation to your hands, the more difficult the exercise becomes.

This exercise can also be done using a railing, a thin tree trunk, the end of a bike rack, a street sign, a balcony support, a light pole, or any kind of pole that's rooted firmly in the ground. I can always find something to do Let Me In's on no matter where I am. All you really need is something firm to hold onto, about waist high, either vertical or horizontal—something that allows you put your feet under or around it. Get creative. You can do it with or without a towel, or even just a thick rope with knots tied in the ends so your hands won't slip off.

Yet another thing you can do to increase the resistance is to lower your hand level, or even prop your feet up on something off the ground. For instance, I happen to have a lattice balustrade surrounding the deck of my apartment building. I put my hand on the top railing—which is waist high—and then I hook my feet into the lattice, about ten inches off the ground, then lean back, sticking my butt out as far as possible, and start cranking these out. The fact is, there's myriad different ways to do Let Me Ins, but do yourself a favor and start with the basics. There's simply nothing better to develop every muscle in your back and biceps.

Ready to kick it up a notch? Try doing Let Me Ins one arm at a time! This'll make a real difference in your forearm, biceps, and lat strength. There are many ways to do this, and different advantages to each of them. Gripping both ends of a towel wrapped around both door knobs is great for increasing grip and forearm strength, as is gripping any edge of a protruding door frame. You can also use any kind of pipe or pole rooted in the ground, or even a thin tree trunk. Just straddle it with your feet as you would normally. Banisters or waist-high Pull Up bars work great too. You can also attach an olympic ring to just about anything and use that. The first time I did these one-handed, I bent a coat hanger so that it looped around the door knobs on both sides of the door, then I wrapped a small towel around the "handle" for a softer grip. This can also be accomplished by looping a strap or rope around the knobs or a tree or railing or pole of any kind anywhere.

Let Me Up's

lats, biceps, forearms, rear deltoids (2-4)

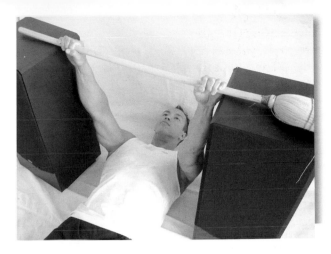

Lie on your back underneath anything that is stable enough for you to pull yourself up with, such as a desk, table, or some type of pole supported by two surfaces (more on this later). It should be just beyond arm's reach above you (about waist high if you are standing). It's okay if the surface is a bit closer than arm's length, but it's not ideal because it will restrict your movement a little.

Lie so that your chest is directly under the thing that you are going to use to pull yourself up on. Reach up and grab the bar or surface with your hands as close to shoulder-width apart as possible, your palms facing your feet.

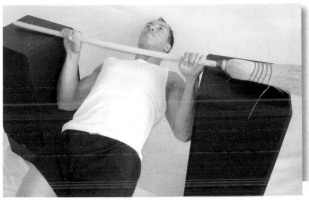

Keeping your body in a rigid line, from your ankles to your shoulders, pull your chest up to the bar or surface, squeezing your shoulder blades together. Only your heels should be touching the ground. Slowly lower yourself back down without letting go of the surface, really stretching out your back and arms at the bottom.

Variations: Keeping your knees bent with your feet flat on the ground, closer to the rest of your body, will make this movement easier.

A wider grip will concentrate more on your lats and a narrower grip on your biceps.

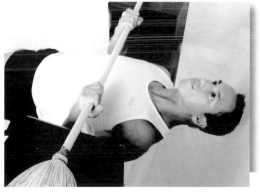

You can do these over- or under-handed, or by using a side grip. Doing them over-handed—either holding a bar or onto the end of a table so that your palms are facing your feet—places more emphasis on the outsides of your forearms (extensors). Doing them with a side grip so that your palms are facing in toward your body—for example, lying beneath a table and holding onto opposite sides of it—will place even more emphasis on the outsides of your forearms. While executing these with a "Reverse Grip"—under-handed like in the photo to the left, will shift the focus to the insides of your forearms (flexors).

Ready to kick it up a notch? Putting your feet up on something like a small table or chair really makes a difference here. Just be sure to keep your back straight, and only bend your hips and legs slightly if you have to in order to complete the motion.

You can also keep one leg in the air during a set to work your quad and abs more, as well as working your glutes and hamstrings since the one leg that is on a surface has to push down in order to keep your body straight during the exercise.

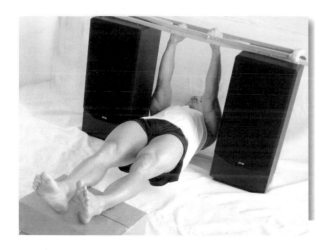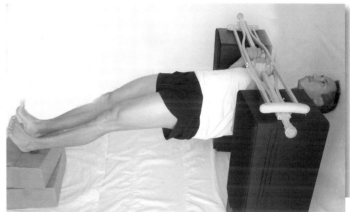

Finding something to do Let Me Ups on:

Look around your home and be creative. I first started doing these by laying a sturdy broom across the tops of two tall stereo speakers, as shown. You can also use a mop or any pole that won't break. You only need to lay it across two even surfaces high enough that the pole is higher than your arm's length above the floor: chairs, tables, file cabinets, you name it. Unless you have a very strong pole, place the two even surfaces just barely wider than shoulder-width apart. Be sure the pole is steady and will not slide one way or the other. (If you need to, if your surfaces are wooden, you can put two small nails around the broomstick on each surface to hold it in place, then, if you want, just remove the nails when you're done and put them aside for the next time.)

  Got an old pair of crutches? Lay them across the two surfaces facing opposite ways so that the handles are about a foot apart and above your chest and get to work! Crutches are absolutely ideal tools for this exercise.

  Keep in mind, you don't even need any kind of pole though. You can use a table or desk as well. This is what I do while on the road and training in a hotel room. Lie with your back on the ground under a table high enough that it's at least arms-length away from you. Your chest should be under the end of the table, and your head poking out looking at the ceiling. Then, just reach up and grab the edge. Just as described above, keeping your heels fixed on the ground, pull yourself up until your chest touches the bottom of the table. Lower yourself slowly until your arms are straight and you can really feel the stretch in your back. If the table's not too wide, you can also grab opposite ends of the table and pull yourself up. You can even do these underhanded by reversing your position under the table—in other words, lie so that your head is under the table and your body and legs protruding out from underneath it. Just reach up and grab the end of the table underhanded and get going!

  Lastly, you don't need it, but if you want, you can buy a Pull Up bar on Amazon.com for less than $20 that will allow you to do both Pull Ups and Let Me Ups in a doorway. Most Pull Up bars come with two pairs of mounts that you put at different heights. Mount one pair at the ideal height for Pull Ups and the other pair at the proper height for Let Me Ups, about waist-high. You can then also use this bar for Let Me In's if you want.

Pull Ups
lats, biceps, forearms (2-4)

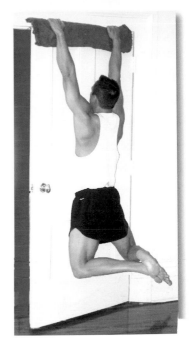

The simplest way to always be able to do Pull Ups, no matter where in the world you are, is do DOOR PULL UPS. Open the door halfway and lay a towel, t-shirt, or cloth over the top. If the towel is not big enough to keep the door from swinging shut, wedge a doorstop, another towel, or something else underneath the door or over one of the hinges. Face the door, place your hands shoulder-width apart on the cloth over the door, and bend your knees, letting your body hang along the door. Pull yourself up against the door until your chin is over the top. Lower yourself slowly until your elbows are straight, really feeling the stretch in your back and arms at the bottom of the movement. Door Pulls have the advantage of making Pull Ups more difficult by not allowing you to swing or kick your legs, and providing extra resistance from the slight friction of your upper thighs being dragged up the door.

Alternatives to using a door: Of course, you can also do this same exercise using a Pull Up bar. A Pull Up bar is a small, removable, and inexpensive piece of equipment that will provide great development for your lats, biceps and forearms. They can also be found in many parks. You can even use a jungle gym.

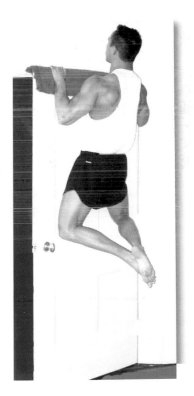

Another great method is to find a tree branch thick enough to support your weight, but thin enough to grasp in both hands. Grab it from either side, hands close together, your palms facing opposite directions, and pull yourself up until your chest touches the branch. Just switch which hand is closer to your head every other set. You can use this side grip variation on a Pull Up bar too. It really strengthens your biceps and forearms.

Or you can use just about any kind of ledge such as a high stable shelf or even a set of stairs that don't have the vertical portion of the steps but only the horizontal one that you actually step on. These can be found at many apartment complexes and motels, among other places. Standing underneath them, grab onto a stair high enough so your feet are off the ground, or bend your knees while holding a lower stair. Again, pull yourself up until your chest touches the stair with your hands on it.

Variations: Can't do a Pull Up yet? Use a surface, such as a chair, to put your feet on behind you, with knees bent, so you can use your legs to assist yourself throughout the movement. After you've done this for a while, or if this is too easy, try jumping to the top of the Pull Up position and concentrate on the negative movement by lowering yourself slowly in a very controlled manner. Keep at it until you build enough strength to pull yourself up without assistance.

As with Let Me Up's, a wider Pull Up grip will concentrate on your lats and a narrower grip more on your biceps. You can do these over- or under-handed, with the underhand grip—palms facing you—placing more emphasis on your insides of your forearms (flexors).

Ready to kick it up a notch? To make Pull Ups harder, wear a weighted backpack. You need very little weight to make this exercise a lot more difficult. Or pull yourself up until your sternum is touching the bar, and hold it for a few seconds before lowering yourself.

Towel Curls

biceps, forearms (2-4)

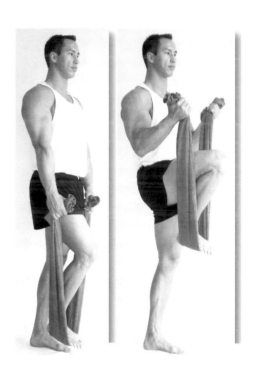

This one's as simple as it is effective. Unlike with weights, you'll be providing your arms with the perfect amount of resistance throughout the entire set.

Stand with your back against a wall for balance. Holding each end of a regular-sized beach or bath towel, raise one leg (it doesn't matter which one) just enough to loop the towel under your foot. Using your leg to provide resistance to your arms, pull up on the towel until you can't go any higher, usually until your forearms are at about a 30-degree angle with your upper arms. The movement should take 5 seconds—count them off. Then 5 seconds to force your hands back down by applying more pressure to the towel with your foot. Only your forearms should move. You elbows should stay fixed by your side and your upper arms perpendicular to the floor. Five reps is all you need to do, no matter your strength, so long as you're giving it maximum effort throughout the entire set.

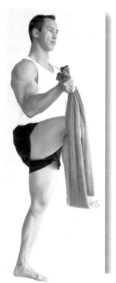

It may take a set or two to get accustomed to using your own body to fight against itself. Of course, your biceps are no match for your legs. Just remember to pull up on the towel as hard as you possibly can, as if you're trying to tear it! (Don't worry, you won't.) And just let your leg move up and down slowly at the same time.

Variation: Do them one-handed.

Ledge Curls
biceps, forearms (2-4)

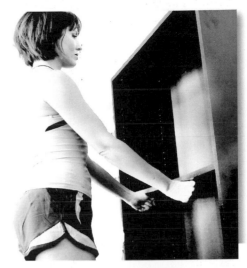

I love these. It's the same as doing Towel Curls in that you make your body fight against itself, only with Ledge Curls you use your back instead of your leg.

Stand, feet shoulder-width apart, in front of anything horizontal, about waist high, stable and fixed, that you can fit your hands under: a staircase railing, balcony railing, strong shelf, drawer, protruding mantle, window-sill, or kitchen counter will all do the trick. Look around and be creative. Just be sure whatever you use is not actually going to budge. It must be stronger, or heavier, than you.

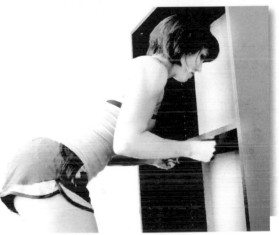

Put your open hands, palms up, under the protruding surface, or in the case of a railing, just grip it as you would a barbell. Your arms should be straight (even if you have to lean back a bit). Try to pull the thing up. Literally try to rip it out of the ground or wall or whatever it's attached to. As you're doing this, slowly bend forward at the waist, keeping your back straight, only bending at the waist and elbows, until your chest or chin touches the thing you're pulling against.

Then slowly reverse the motion, leaning back until you are standing up straight again. Again, try to break the thing. Keep your elbows locked in place, down at the side of your body. Only your hips and elbows should bend. Never stop pulling with your arms, but instead go right into another rep. Each positive and negative movement should take 5 seconds, and 5 reps is all you need to really blast your biceps. I personally love doing these at the end of a Pull workout, to finish off my biceps.

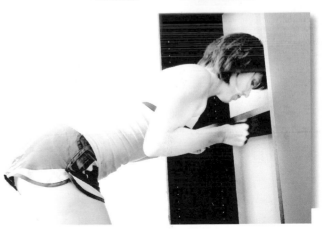

Variation: You can also do these with a side-grip, focusing more attention on the outsides of your forearms, much like hammer curls. Just make fists beneath the ledge you are pull-ing against so that your thumbs and index fingers are facing up and touching the ledge, like in the pictures. If you have ac-cess to a horizontal staircase railing or banister with spindles, just grip a spindle at its top in each hand, and go to work, literally trying to rip up the railing as you do the exercise.

Curls

biceps, forearms (1-4)

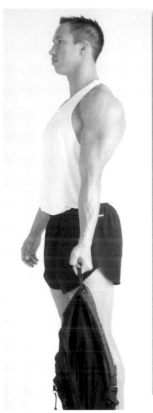
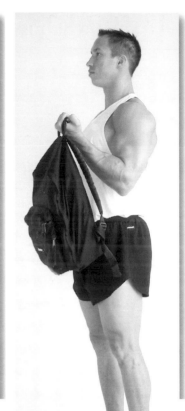

Just because you don't have dumbbells doesn't mean you can't do Curls. Curls can be done with just about anything, such as jugs of milk or water, grocery bags filled with things, or my favorite: a backpack filled with something heavy—books, magazines, newspapers, cans of food, recycled bottles filled with water, rocks, sand, just about anything. Add things until you have the perfect weight and hold the top strap of the backpack. You can even make a proper handle out of it if you like: Just brake off a few inches of a stick that's the proper width for a handle and use duct tape or electrical tape to fasten it to the back pack's top handle. See Appendix 1 for a demonstration.

Stand with your feet shoulder-width apart and good posture—your chest out with your shoulders back and down. Keep your elbow locked in place on the side of your body, just above your hip, and curl the weight toward your shoulder.

Variation: Doing curls with your palms facing down will make them quite a bit more difficult and emphasize the outsides of your forearms (extensors) more.

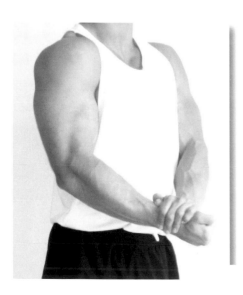

Isometric Curls require no equipment at all. Grasp the wrist of your working arm with your other hand and push down on it so hard that you can barely raise your arm as you would with any other kind of curl. You are using the triceps of one arm to work against the biceps and forearm muscles of your other arm.

Forearm Curls

forearms (duh) (1-4)

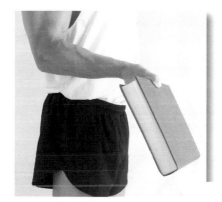

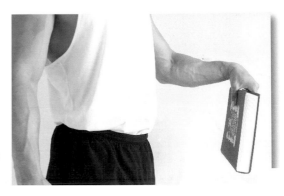

Pick up any object that you can grip easily, like a phone book, bottle of water or juice, or just a can of soup. The longer and heavier the object—like a big hardback book or a closed laptop computer—the harder this exercise becomes.

Hold your forearm out so that it is parallel to the ground. Hold your palm up, facing the ceiling, in order to work the insides of your forearms (flexors). If your palm is down, facing the floor, you'll work the outside of your forearms (extensors). Move the object up and down using only your wrist, pausing for a second at the top. Your forearm should always stay parallel to the ground and at a 90-degree angle with your upper arm.

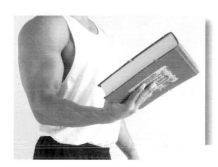

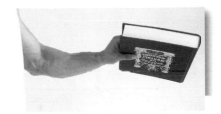

You can, of course, exercise both forearms at the same time—by gripping two similar objects or one larger object—or focus on just one at a time, your choice.

Variation: A great way to tone both sides of your forearm at the same time, while increasing your grip strength, is to hold the object straight out and turn it over, back and forth, back and forth. Sometimes I do this after a regular set of Forearm Curls.

The Claw

hands and forearms (1)

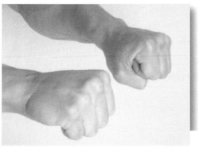

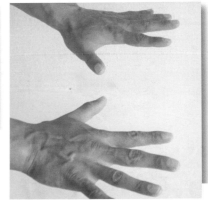

As effective as it is simple. Repeatedly open and close your hands as tightly and quickly as possible. Hold them open, fingers spread wide as possible, for half a second, then shut them with lightning speed, and clench them closed for half a second, before again opening them as fast as possible. 50 - 100 should do the trick.

LEG & GLUTE
Exercises

I'll start you out easy here with some exercises for your hamstrings and glutes, including movements that might make your butt defy gravity, like Bam Bams. I move on to quad and squatting exercises—from starting with your back resting against a wall to Sumo and Sissy Squats and working up to unassisted One-Legged Squats and Pistols, the greatest exercise for overall leg strength and balance. I complement these with movements that build explosive power like Star Jumpers and Iron Mikes. I'll explain how to vary any thigh exercise slightly to focus on different muscles in your quads, which will shape your legs accordingly. And finally, I'll show you how to most effectively work all your calf muscles.

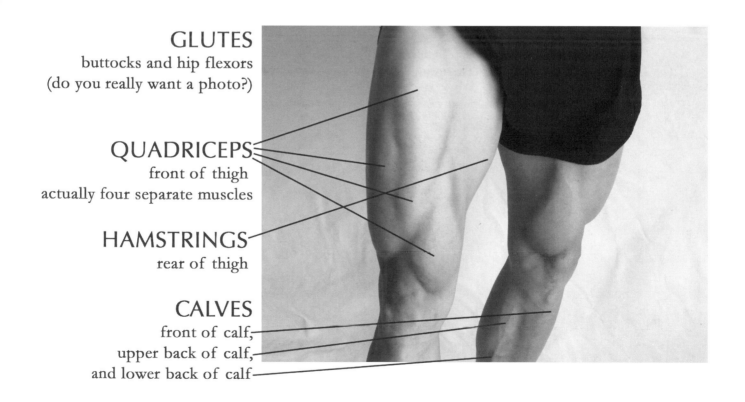

GLUTES
buttocks and hip flexors
(do you really want a photo?)

QUADRICEPS
front of thigh
actually four separate muscles

HAMSTRINGS
rear of thigh

CALVES
front of calf,
upper back of calf,
and lower back of calf

Good Mornings

glutes, hamstrings, lower back (1)

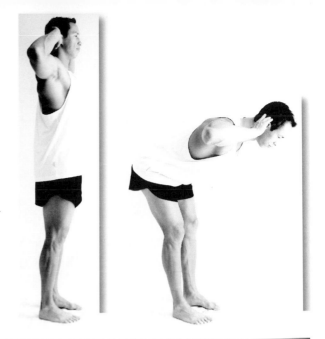

Stand with your feet shoulder-width apart and your hands behind your head. Then bow down, bending only at the waist, keeping your back arched (chest and butt out), and your legs almost straight.

You should feel tension in the backs of your legs. Bend over until you can't anymore, always maintaining an arch in your back. Do not slope your shoulders downward, but keep them back, chest out, throughout the movement. Your waist is the only thing that should bend.

Return to the starting position.

Hooya!

Not So Good Mornings

Hey, even I gotta take a break sometimes.

I flew to New Orleans for a long weekend to do some of the photos you see here. We shot them in a studio in the famed French Quarter. After two exhausting days, my co writer, Joshua Clark, and I decided to hit the street in search of a few drinks. En route we came across a couple of young guys testing their jumping skills by trying to reach a bar sign hanging from a tall balcony. It must have been eight or nine feet up. After a few luckless attempts they moved on. Of course, when I was under the sign I couldn't resist testing my "ups" as well, and to my surprise, I tapped the sign. We continued on to the bar and found the same fellas having a beer there. After chatting with them awhile, feeling froggy, I decided to bet them that I could jump without taking a step and land flat-footed on top of the bar. The wager: A round of Irish Car Bombs. (A shot of half Jameson whiskey, half Bailey's, dropped into a pint of Guinness and chugged.)

I'm not quite sure why I thought this was a good idea, and I'd never tried it before, but we waited until the bartendress was turned the other way and— Luckily, the bet worked in our favor. I pulled it off, then leaped down before she saw me. Then it went double or nothing, and I landed it again. Finally, one of the young guys we'd challenged decided to give it a whirl himself, proclaiming to a bunch of nearby ladies that it was no big deal. He jumped, but didn't quite make it. And just as the bartender turned around, he got his foot caught on the bar's underside, and groping for something to break his fall straight backwards, he swiped every glass off the bar onto the floor in a series of thunderous crashes.

That's when we got kicked out and found another bar to try our stupid human trick. Round after round we went from bar to bar like a traveling circus with its freak show hustling for Irish Car Bombs. I'm proud to say that my greatest conquest was a bar that came to my chest, with me being 5'11", and a belly weighed down with near a dozen Car Bombs. For some reason I also thought it would be funny to jump down—not back to where I had been standing—but on the other side, behind the bar… Only it wasn't so funny when the bartender turned around and a person had suddenly, magically materialized behind her. She couldn't figure out how I had done it, but she knew the solution: "Get out!"

It goes without saying that the next morning's photo shoot was a bit painful. And the only reason I'm not grimacing in a few of these photos is because of the photographer's constant reminders. I felt like a little kid who hates getting his portrait taken, over and over and over again…

Good morning? *Good night!*

Dirty Dogs

glutes, lower back, hip flexors (1)

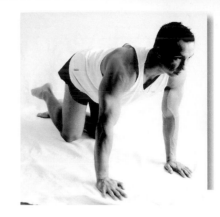

Get down on all fours. Your hands should be shoulder-width apart, your back straight and your knees bent at 90-degree angles.

Keeping your knee bent at 90 degrees, swing your right leg out to the side as high as possible. Hold this peak position and contract your glutes for three seconds. Now you know how this one got its name. Keep your hips squared in a fixed position throughout the movement. Only your one leg should move. And remember: fight the urge to bend your knee more—be sure to keep it fixed at 90 degrees. Then bring your leg back down to the starting position, and repeat the movement with your left leg.

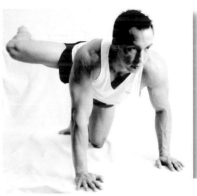

Ready to kick it up a notch? Don't alternate legs, but rather do reps continually on one leg at a time until it's exhausted, then switch to the other leg.

Mule Kick

hamstrings, glutes, lower back (1)

Get down on your hands and knees with your hands shoulder-width apart, back straight and knees bent at a 90-degree angle (just like Dirty Dogs).

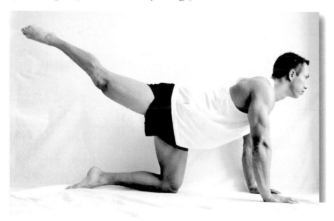

Slowly kick your right leg straight back and up as high as possible, keeping your hips fixed squarely in place. Hold this peak position for five seconds, then bring your leg back down to the starting position. Then do the same with your left leg.

Ready to kick it up a notch? Don't alternate legs, but rather do reps continually on one leg at a time until it burns like hell, then switch to the other.

Standing Side Leg Lift

glutes, hip flexors, lower back (1)

Stand with your feet hip distance apart, holding onto a chair or desk lightly for balance. In a slow and controlled manner, lift your right leg out to the side, keeping your hip, knee, ankle and toes all in alignment, and your foot flexed. Raise your right leg until it is about 45 degrees out to the side. Squeeze your glutes and hold this peak position for two seconds. Then slowly lower your leg back down without relaxing your glutes.

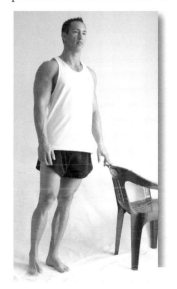 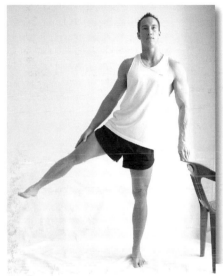

Be sure to keep the standing leg slightly bent. Also, make sure the toes and knee of the leg you are lifting face forward throughout the movement. The key here is to stay standing absolutely straight and keep your shoulders and hips stable, squared and facing forward. And, remember, don't stick your butt back at all in the top of the movement.

Standing Leg Curls

glutes, hamstrings (1)

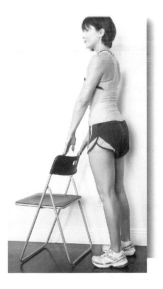 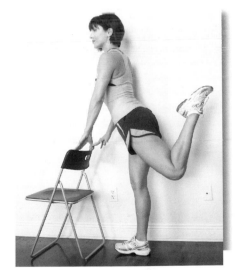

Stand with your feet shoulder-width apart with your hands lightly holding something in front of you for balance. Raise your right leg back and up as high as possible behind you. Curl your right heel in toward your butt. Hold for three seconds, really squeezing it, then bring your leg back down to the ground, and repeat, until it's time to switch to the other leg.

One-Legged Romanian Dead Lifts

hamstrings, lower back, balance (2)

Stand upright with your feet together. Keep your back as straight as possible and reach down with your right arm until you have touched the ground in front of your left foot, raising your right leg straight behind you as you lower your upper body. Your knees should remain straight throughout the motion but not quite locked.

Return to the upright position and then reach down and touch the ground in front of your left foot, again, but with your left hand this time. You have completed one rep after you have touched the ground with both hands. When you are done with your left leg, switch to your right.

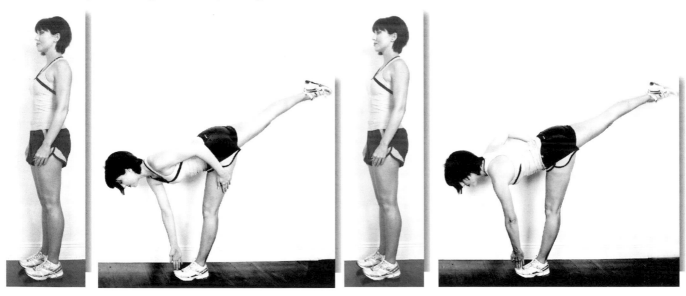

Ready to Kick it up a Notch? Do it on a soft surface like a pillow or couch cushion that challenges your balance. You can also wear a weighted backpack. Or finish each repetition with a jump. The Romanian Dead Lift and jump should be one fluid motion. Land on both legs. Try jumping on an object if you're strong enough!

Hip Extensions

glutes, hamstrings, lower back (2-3)

Lie flat on your back with your arms at your side and your heels resting on an elevated platform such as a chair. Your knees should be bent at about a 90-degree angle. Now, using only your legs, push your hips upward as high as you can. Your thighs should be in a straight line with your back. Hold this peak position for a two second contraction, really squeezing your hamstrings and glutes. Then slowly lower your hips back to the starting position.

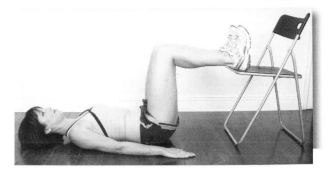

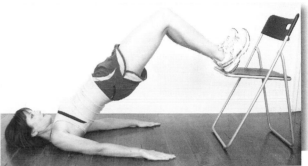

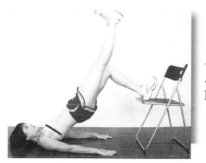

Ready to kick it up a notch? Do this exercise one leg at a time.

King of the Klutz

calves, quads, hamstrings, hip flexors, and balance (1-4)

Stand on one leg. Close your eyes.

That's it. Seriously. Think it's funny? See how long you can do it for.

Great party trick: Bet your buddy or significant other they can't do it for one minute.

Ready to kick it up a notch? Once you can do that for a minute with no problem, try doing it with your eyes open, but your head back, looking at the ceiling straight above you. And once you've conquered that for a minute, try doing it while looking up and keeping your eyes closed.

Next, try standing on a thick pillow or other soft surface, head back, eyes closed. And when you've got that down, try it on a curved surface like a log!

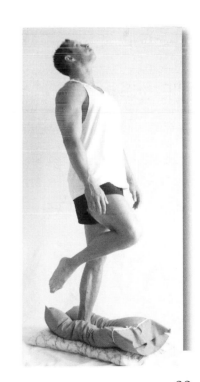

Bam Bams

glutes (2)

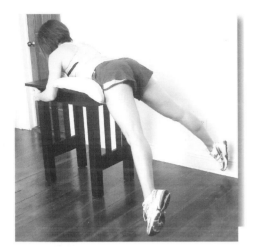

If you get into the habit of doing these after you're done with Lunges or Squats it shouldn't be long until it looks like your rear end skipped physics class the day they taught gravity.

Lie belly down on the corner of a bed (or on the edge of a large stable surface like a dinner table, coffee table or desk) so that the corner is below your pelvis and your entire legs are hanging off the bed to either side of the corner. If you wish, you can place a pillow underneath your pelvis for added comfort. Stabilize yourself by holding onto different sides of the bed or table.

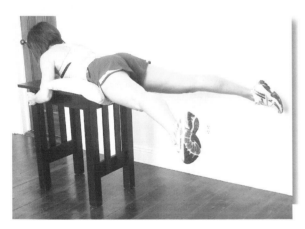

Spread your legs as wide as possible, then, with your knees only very slightly bent, lift your legs off the ground as high as possible.

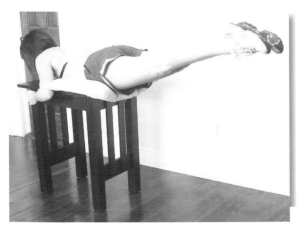

Bring them together until your heels lightly touch, keeping your knees only slightly bent. Your feet should create a crescent arc through the air as you bring them up as high as you can. Be sure to really squeeze your glutes at the top of the movement, and hold it for three seconds. Then slowly lower your legs back to the floor as you spread them wide at the same time. A few sets of ten reps should do the trick.

YOU ARE YOUR OWN GYM

Ham Sandwich

hamstrings, and explosive power in your chest and shoulders (4)

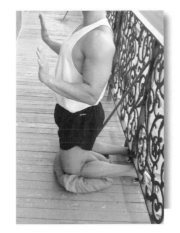

Kneel on a pillow and hook your heels under something fixed to the ground like the bottom of a railing balustrade (as in the pictures) or something heavy like a couch, or, if you have a partner, have them hold your ankles down.

Start with your body upright and keep your back straight.

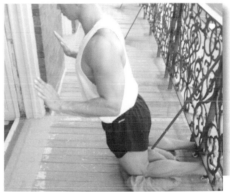

Only bending at your knees, let yourself have a controlled fall, face first, to the ground, breaking the fall with your hands in a slow, controlled manner. Only bend at the knees. Your hips should not bend at all. Your back should stay in a straight line with your thighs.

Control is the key here. *Use your hamstrings to slow your fall down as much as possible*, then when you put your hands out let your fingers brace your weight first for a split second before your weight falls on your palms. It should make almost no noise when your hands hit the ground, because you are not slamming them into the ground. Then let your chest touch the ground as though you were doing a Push Up.

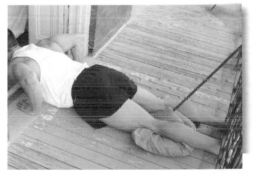

Explode back up like you're doing a Bouncing Push Up, but use your hamstrings as much as possible.

After your fingers leave the ground, use only your hamstrings to bring your body back to the full and upright position.

Ready to kick it up a notch? Doing these one-handed really forces you to use your hamstrings to the max, and depend much less on your arm muscles to slow you down and push yourself back up. Try using your arm less and less, until you're hardly pushing at all. Eventually you can try doing them without your hands at all!

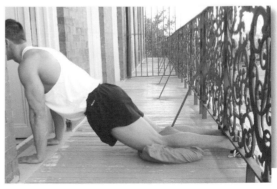

SQUATS

All squatting exercises are usually done with your toes pointing straight forward, or slightly pointing out, as your feet are when you walk. You can adjust any squatting exercise to focus more attention on your *vastus medialis* (the teardrop-shaped muscle that protrudes just above the inside of each knee and runs about a third of the length of the thigh—the one that wearing shorts really shows off) by keeping your toes pointed further out than 30 degrees from straight ahead. Alternatively, doing any squatting exercise with your toes pointed inward will emphasize your *vastus lateralis* (a.k.a. the *look-fabulous-in-slim-jeans-or-a-bathing-suit* muscle) which creates the curve, or "sweep" of your outer thigh.

Squats

quads, hamstrings, glutes, lower back, and hip flexors (1-4)

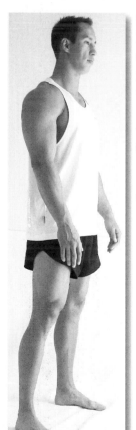

Stand with your feet shoulder-width apart. With your head up and eyes forward, bend your knees until your butt is a couple inches above the floor. Lean your upper body slowly forward as you go down, until your shoulders are out over your knees. But be sure your knees do not protrude past your toes (this can lead to knee pains). Then, keeping your heels on the floor, slowly stand again using only your legs to lift you.

At first, try practicing these facing a wall, with your toes 4 – 6 inches from the wall. This is a great way of correcting technique by ensuring that your knees are not going too far forward.

Variations: If going into a full squat is too difficult at first, lower yourself only as far as you can, until you develop the strength and flexibility needed to lower your body all the way down.

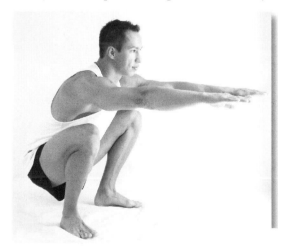

If you need to, you can hold onto something about waist-high to steady yourself and help push yourself back up.

If you place your feet closer together (and/or point your toes outward) this exercise will focus more on the muscles of your inner thighs; while with your legs further apart than shoulder-width (and/or your toes straight ahead or inward), it will put more emphasis on your outer thighs.

Ready to kick it up a notch? Load up a backpack or even have a training partner, girlfriend, wife, or child sit on your shoulders.

Invisible Chair

quadriceps, hamstrings, glutes (1)

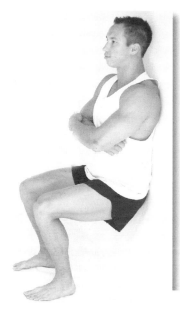

Stand with your back to a wall.

Move your feet away from the wall, but keep your hips and back against the wall so that the wall is supporting you.

Bending at the knees, lower your body until your thighs are parallel to the ground. Your knees should be directly above your feet and be bent at 90 degrees.

Simply hold this position for as long as you can.

Ready to kick it up a notch? Try holding some weight.

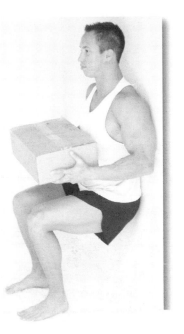

Wall Squat

quadriceps, hamstrings, glutes (1)

Wearing a t-shirt, stand up with your back against a smooth wall, door or doorway. Move both your feet one step forward, but keep your hips and back against the wall so that the wall is supporting you. Then, bending at the knees, slowly lower your body until your thighs are parallel to the ground. If your feet are in the correct place, your knees should be directly above your feet and be bent at 90 degrees. Keeping your butt and back against the wall, and your feet locked in place, push yourself up until your legs are straight again.

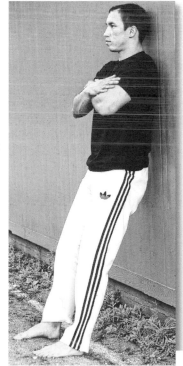

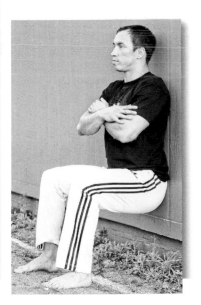

Beat Your Boots

hamstrings, quads (2)

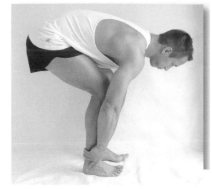

This was a favorite remedial exercise to correct poor performance at the Army's Parachutist Course. You won't think this one's so silly after you do 30 of them.

Standing with your legs together, bend down and grab your ankles. Keep your legs as straight as you can comfortably hold them. Then bend your knees until your butt touches your hands on your ankles. Keeping your hands on your ankles, lift your butt upwards, again straightening your knees as much as you can comfortably.

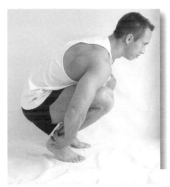

Sumo Squat

hamstrings, quadriceps, glutes (1)

Take a wide stance with your toes pointed out. While keeping your back straight, swing your arms out in front of you and drop your hips until your thighs are parallel to the ground.

Push yourself back up to the start position, really squeezing your glutes tightly at the top. Hold the contraction at the top of the movement for a couple of seconds.

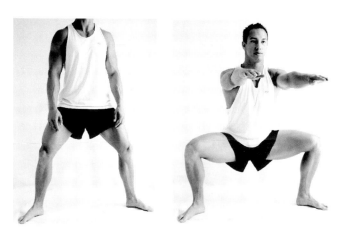

Variation: Try it on your toes.

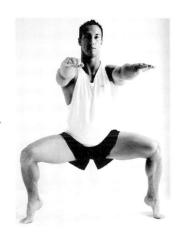

Advanced Sumo Squat

hamstrings, quadriceps, glutes (2-4)

A 6-count movement

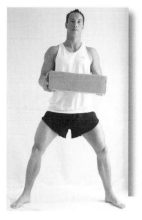

Standing with your feet shoulder-width apart, hold some sort of weight in both hands in front of your waist with your elbows bent at a 90-degree angle. It can be anything at all—a bag filled with something, a water jug or two, phone books, a box… you get the idea.

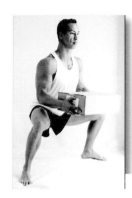

Perform a Sumo Squat (Count 1).

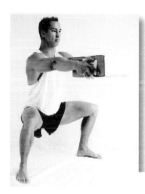

At the bottom, bring the weight straight out in front of you until your arms are straight (2).

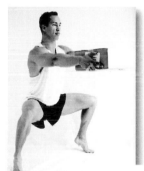

Raise up on your toes (3).

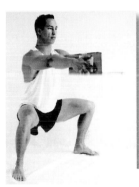

Bring your heels back down (4).

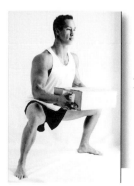

Bring your arms back in (5).

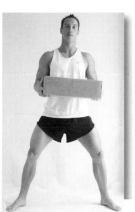

Stand up and squeeze those glutes at the top (6)!

Lunges

quadriceps, glutes, with secondary focus on the hamstrings and hip flexors (1-4)

Stand with your feet together, toes pointed straight ahead. Take a big step forward with your left foot, bending your knees and lowering your hips until your trailing right knee almost touches the ground. Both knees should be bent to 90 degrees at this point. Your front left knee should be directly over your foot but not past your toes.

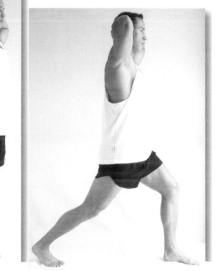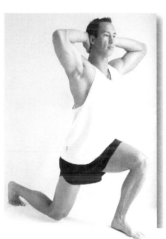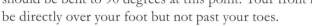

Being sure to keep your head up and back straight throughout the exercise, push up with your left leg, and step back to the starting position. Do not lock your knees.

Repeat the movement with the other foot.

Variations: To make things a bit easier, stand with your legs already apart, as though you were in mid-stride. If you need to, hold onto a chair or other stable surface for balance. With your weight evenly distributed over each foot, slowly lower your hips until both knees are at 90-degree angles and your trailing knee almost touches the floor. Again, do not let your front knee extend over your toes. Push through the heel on the front foot, squeeze your glutes and raise yourself back up to the starting position without locking your knees.

You can also make these easier by lunging onto a step or low table that's in front of you. Then work your way up to being able to do them on the ground.

If you've got space, you can even do "Walking Lunges" by stepping forward with your left foot as described above, but instead of bringing your left foot back to the starting position, you bring your right foot up to your left one. Then take a step forward with your right foot, and repeat the motion. Keep "walking" until you can't anymore.

Back Lunges are done by taking a big step backward, instead of forward. Again, bend your knees and lower your hips until your trailing knee almost touches the ground. Then push yourself back up with your front foot, and step forward so that your feet are together again.

Ready to kick it up a notch? Try holding water jugs or sandbags or anything else you can get your hands on. Just hold them straight down to either side of you. Or else load up a backpack and put it on. Even a little extra weight will make it a lot more difficult to balance and work your muscles all the harder. You can also do "Overhead Lunges" by holding the objects or a single object like a weighted backpack overhead with your elbows locked out straight.

YOU ARE YOUR OWN GYM

Side Lunges

quadriceps, glutes, hip flexors, hamstrings (2-4)

Stand upright with your feet slightly apart and your hands in front of your legs. Take a wide step to the side with your left foot, your toes pointing slightly outward. As your left foot comes in contact with the ground, shift your weight onto it.

Keeping your upper body fixed and vertical and your abs contracted, lower your hips straight down. Your right leg should stay straight. Your upper body should move forward only slightly, and your bottom should stick out behind you. Your left knee should not move forward at all. Keep your left shin vertical and come down until your left thigh is parallel to the ground. Keep your head up and your back straight throughout the movement. Hold the tension in your left leg for two seconds, then raise your body straight up by pushing against the floor with your left heel, and return to the starting position.

You should be able to execute the entire movement without losing balance. If you loose balance, you just need to start out taking a more narrow step to the side. When you've done all the repetitions you can with your left leg, switch to your right leg. This is one of the few movements that work side-to-side motion, and a great way to develop the strength needed to do One-Legged Squats.

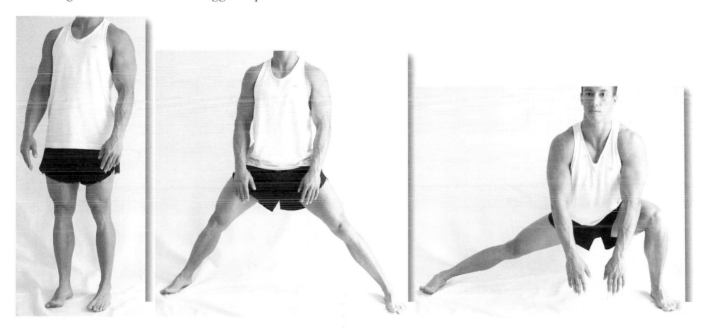

Variation: You can also do Side Lunges keeping your feet fixed in the wide stance, as in the middle photograph. Simply do not return your feet to the starting position, but instead continue squatting down on each leg, one at a time, using the posture described above, until you've exhausted both legs and you're finished with your set.

Ready to kick it up a notch? Put on a backpack filled with books or water bottles or rocks. It makes a huge difference.

Iron Mikes

quadriceps, glutes, hip flexors, hamstrings, and balance (3)

Start out in the bottom position of a regular Lunge. Your left foot should be planted firmly on the ground in front of you. Your left knee should be bent at 90 degrees directly over your left foot. Your right leg should be behind you, also bent at 90 degrees, and your right knee a couple inches above the ground. Keep your back straight, your head upright, and your shoulders squared throughout the movement.

From this position, pushing primarily off your front foot, spring into the air high enough to switch legs and land so that your left leg is back and your right leg is forward, both at 90 degrees. Of course, you will not land directly in this position, but you will drop into it quickly after your feet make contact with the ground. Repeat until you can no longer make it off the ground.

The first few times you try Iron Mikes you may find it difficult to balance, but that's what makes the exercise so great. Your stabilizing muscles will catch on real quick and start toning up.

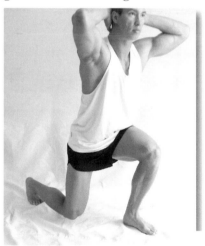 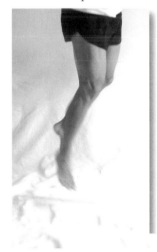 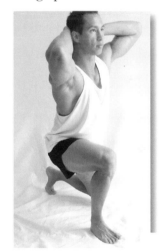

Variation: Try staying up on your toes through the movement. This'll not only develop your calves but it'll kick your leg strength and balance up a notch as well.

Toyotas

quadriceps, glutes, hip flexors, hamstrings, calves (1)

Like the following exercise, Star Jumpers, but a little more basic: Go into a full Squat, then place your palms on the ground, and jump as high as possible into the air while simply shooting your hands straight up overhead. Land as softly as possible and repeat.

Star Jumpers

quadriceps, glutes, hip flexors, hamstrings, calves (2)

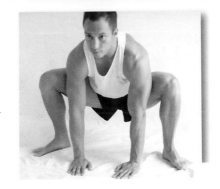

This literal ass smoker is handed out like candy at the Army's Special Forces selection course.

Start in the bottom Sumo Squat position. Your feet should be more than shoulder-width apart, planted firmly on the ground, toes pointing outward, your butt a few inches off the ground, back straight, shoulders squared, head up, and your hands touching the ground between your feet. Then explode into the air, stretching your arms and legs out as wide as possible. And drop back down into the starting position.

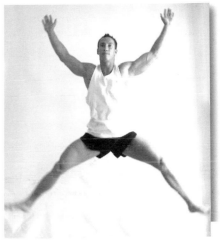

Be sure not to land flat on your feet, or worse, your heels. Always cushion your fall back to the earth by landing on your toes for a split second before your heels touch ground as your legs are bending and you return to the starting position, hands on the ground.

Variation: Keeping your heels up off the ground throughout the movement will further develop your calves as well as your balance.

Side Jumps

quadriceps, hamstrings, glutes, hip flexors, calves (2-4)

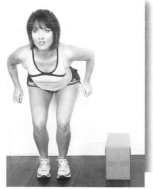
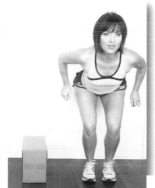

This is a great exercise that builds explosive power and strength. Simply jump back and forth over an object sideways. The object you are jumping over should be on one side of you when starting and on the opposite side when finishing each rep. Start with your legs closer than shoulder-width apart and your toes pointed straight ahead or slightly outward. Try to land with your feet in exactly the same position.

Ready to kick it up a notch? Do it on one leg. Keep going until clearing the object becomes very difficult, then switch legs, then do both feet at once. It's safest to just lay a pillow on the ground, or even two shoes or socks about a foot apart, and just jump from one side of them to the other, rather than using something high like a box that you might trip over during your last few reps.

HIP POWER MOVEMENTS

quadriceps, hamstrings, glutes, hip flexors, lower back, calves (1-4)

Building explosive power is too often the weak point of bodyweight regimens. So here are some more great exercises for just that. These develop your "fast twitch" muscle fibers which are four times bigger than the slow twitch ones.

Box Jumps

Find any object to jump on, such as stairs, a solid box, table, or other platform. Using a shoulder-width stance, go into a quarter to half squat position and explode forcefully onto the object. Be sure to pick your legs up high in order to get as much clearance as possible. Step off the platform and back to the starting position using an alternating backwards lunge. Doing this on stairs, moving up one stair at a time as you build strength, is a great way to measure your progress. Obviously, the higher the object is, the more difficult this exercise becomes. But you don't need to only jump as high as the object. You should always try to jump as high as possible, even if that is higher in the air than the object you're using.

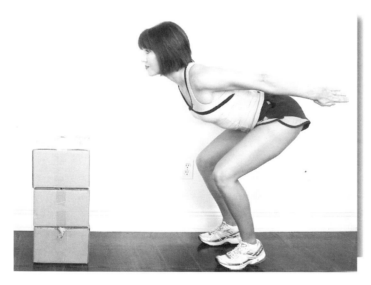
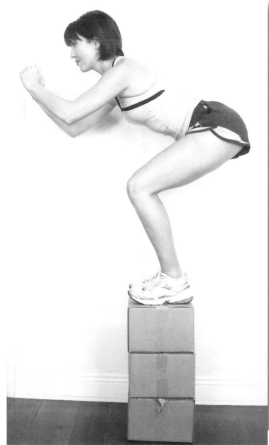

Ready to kick it up a notch? Try it with just one leg at a time! This is simply awesome for not only building strength but balance and coordination too.

Full Squat Jumps

Using a shoulder-width stance, sink your hips until your butt touches your heels, while keeping your heels on the floor. Start slowly and pick up speed throughout the movement until you have exploded through the top and are airborne. Keep your arms tucked into your chest. Again, you should always try to jump as high as possible, even if that is higher in the air than the object you're using.

Half Squat Jumps

Same as Full Squat Jumps, except start with your thighs about parallel to the ground. You'll need to be more forceful off the start.

Quarter Squat Jumps

Start from the standing position, dip down into a quarter squat position with your knees only bent about 45 degrees, and explode into the air.

Depth Jumps

Jump off a platform and immediately jump back on it. The height of the platform should be 6" - 24". Here's the key: The duration of your feet's impact with the ground should be no more than a fraction of a second. If the height of the platform is so high that it causes you to spend more than about a tenth of second, you need to find a lower platform. A few sets of 8 - 12 reps should do the trick.

This is a great exercise for increasing your vertical jump. Depth Jumps train your body to quickly and efficiently reverse energy, which is a key skill when initiating a jump. Definitely not a good choice for beginners, this exercise is high impact and requires fairly high levels of strength.

One-Legged Squat with Jump

Finish a One-Legged Squat with a jump. Land on both legs and repeat.

One-Legged Romanian Dead Lift with Jump

Finish a One-Legged RDL with a jump. Land on both legs and repeat.

Overhead Squats

quads, hamstrings, glutes, hip flexors, lower back, spinal erectors, shoulders (3)

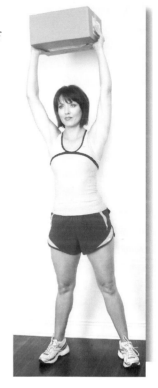

Perform a squat while holding an object, such as a weighted backpack, overhead. The top of your thighs should be parallel to the ground in the bottom position. Your feet should be shoulder-width apart with your toes pointing outward no more than thirty degrees. Your heels should remain on the ground, and your knees should point in the same direction as your index toe.

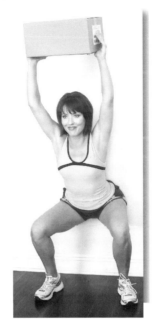

This exercise requires a bit more practice than most because you'll need a good amount of balance and flexibility in order to hold an object overhead while in the bottom of a squat. For added stability, shrug your shoulders as high as possible throughout the movement, lock your elbows, and act as if you were trying to pull the object apart. Begin with a broomstick or a towel—pulling the towel taut—and use a wide grip, if you are unfamiliar with this exercise. As you build flexibility and movement proficiency, use a narrower grip until you are able to hold an item such as a weighted backpack while in the bottom position. Overhead squats are great for developing good squatting technique, shoulder flexibility, and strength in the shoulder girdle.

Squat Thrusts

quads, hamstrings, glutes, lower back, hip flexors, spinal erectors, shoulders, triceps (1-4)

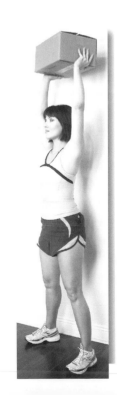

Take any object, such as weighted backpack, and hold it at chest level. Lower yourself into a deep squat, bringing your butt down as far as possible. Remember, don't let your knees go forward past your toes.

Stand up and push the object straight overhead. This should be one fluid movement.

While lowering the object from the overhead position, go into another deep squat. Again, this should be one distinct movement.

Ready to kick it up a notch? Try jumping into the air at the top of the movement! Just be sure to land softly on your toes and go back into a squat.

Bulgarian Split Squat

quadriceps, hamstrings, glutes (2-4)

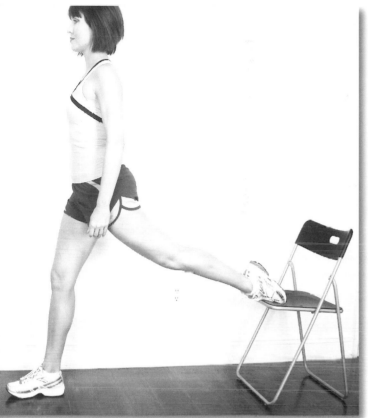

Somewhat similar to a regular Lunge but for one very effective difference: Your back leg is elevated on an object like a chair or bed about two feet behind you. For comfort, you can put a pillow on the chair, and your foot on the pillow. Work on your balance and don't hold onto anything. This is a great exercise which works both legs, but be sure to push mainly off the foot that is on the ground. This is also a great way to lead up to doing One-Legged Squats.

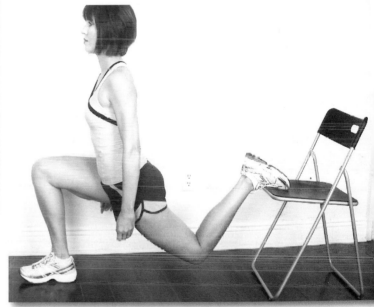

Ready to kick it up a notch? Try wearing a weighted backpack.

For a still more difficult variation, and to work your shoulders at the same time, try holding a weighted backpack overhead with your arms locked out, or press the backpack from your chest to the overhead position and lower it back down while at the bottom of the Split Squat. And once you've mastered those, it's time for…

One-Legged Squats

quads, hamstrings, glutes, lower back and hip flexors (4)

This is probably the world's greatest exercise for strengthening your legs and glutes. It works every component of fitness: strength, coordination, balance, endurance, you name it. And with a little creativity, the variations are endless.

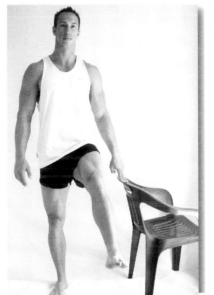

Lift your left leg up and stand on your right leg, holding onto something about waist level, like a chair, lightly for balance, with your head up and back straight.

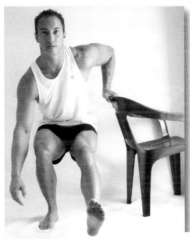

Slowly lower your body, bending at your waist and right knee, until your right thigh is parallel to the floor, and your shoulders are forward past your knees. Keep your left foot off the ground and in front of you. Do not let your right knee extend forward past the toes of your right foot. Be sure to keep your back straight.

Using only your right leg, push yourself back up. Remember, your hand is only holding onto something in order to stabilize you, not to help push your body up. And don't quite lock your knee at the top of the movement.

After you can't do anymore, switch to your left foot.

Variations: To make this exercise easier, use an elevated surface to sit on before standing up, like a low coffee table or a chair. The higher the surface, the easier the exercise gets. Simply lower yourself slowly onto it with one leg, then focus on pushing yourself back up. As you get stronger, use a lower surface, until eventually you can sit on the floor and explode back up on one leg. By that time, a regular One-Legged Squat will be easy as pie.

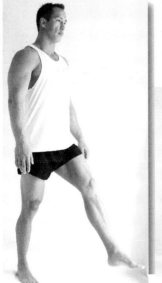

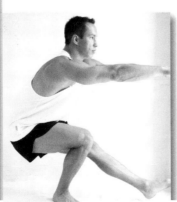

Try One-Legged Squats with your nonworking leg raised off the ground and bent *behind* you. Come down until you lightly touch your nonworking knee to the ground. You'll need to really lean forward when executing this movement, and stick your hands straight out in front of you for balance.

Ready to kick it up a notch? Let go of that chair! Don't hold onto anything, but instead just put your arms out for balance. I don't care how much weight you can pile on your back at the gym's squat rack, this will strengthen your legs and butt like never before, as well as greatly enhance your balance.

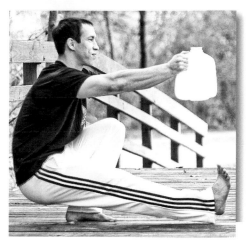

Really ready to kick it up a notch? Do # Pistols. Bring your butt all the way down to the heel of your working foot. Keep the negative movement slow and controlled and then explode back up.

If you lack flexibility in your ankles and hip flexors, try slightly elevating your heel by placing something about the thickness of a flip-flop underneath it.

You can make this still more difficult by holding some kind of weight with both hands in front of your chest, like water jugs or a rock-filled backpack—just use your imagination, and this amazing exercise will never stop making you stronger.

Another great way to do Pistols, especially if you're having trouble with the flexibility required to keep your nonworking leg straight out in front of you, is to do them on a very stable table, desk, kitchen counter or other waist-high platform that can hold your weight. Stand on the platform so that its edge is between your feet, with one foot on the platform near its edge, and the other hanging off it in the air. Your nonworking leg stays in the air, hanging straight down as you perform the Squat with your other leg. Come all the way down until your butt touches the surface. This allows more range of motion than a typical Pistol and is a truly great muscle builder.

To make this exercise harder, and to really build your balance, hold onto your nonworking leg like you're stretching your thigh. Hold the top of your foot behind your butt, so that your nonworking knee is pointing straight down. Now lower yourself with your other leg, until your nonworking knee lightly touches the ground (if you're not on a rug, use a pillow or towel).

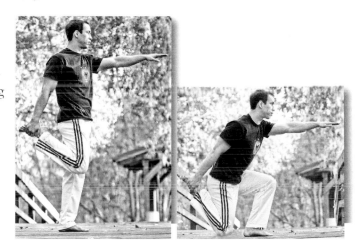

Another method to build great leg power is to pause twice on the way back up. When your thigh is just below parallel to the floor, pause and count out five seconds. Then pause again when your thigh is just above parallel with the floor, again counting slowly to five. Finally, push yourself the rest of the way up. These are your two greatest sticking points, and working on them will bring your thighs to new levels of strength. Try holding a heavy weight to your chest and doing just one rep on each leg.

Yet another great twist to add is to finish your One-Legged Squat with a jump. The squat and the jump should be one fluid motion. Land on your other leg, then do a squat and jump on that leg. Try jumping onto an object like a phone book or something if you can.

Sissy Squats

thighs, hamstrings, glutes (3-4)

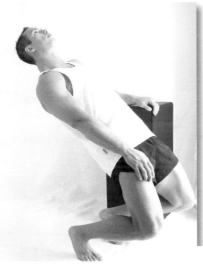

Don't let the name fool you. Believe me, there ain't nothing sissy about these!

Stand with your feet shoulder-width apart, lightly holding onto something about waist level for balance. Bending only at the knees, lower yourself down, leaning back, until your butt touches your heels. You should be up on your toes at this point. The key here is to keep your back and thighs in a straight line throughout the entire movement, not bending at the hips at all.

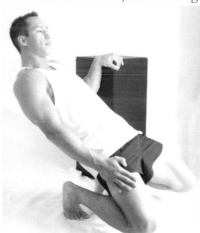

Then, using every muscle from your butt to your calves, again keeping your back and thighs in a straight line, reverse the movement, pushing up until you are standing again.

These closely mimic the same motion as leg extensions, only using more muscles.

Ready to kick it up a notch? You can hold something heavy to your chest with your free hand, or put on a loaded backpack.

Really ready to kick it up a notch? Try doing these one leg at a time! For balance, you'll need to hold lightly onto two things, both about waist-high (like chairs), on either side of you. Keep your nonworking leg straight out in front of you, just barely off the ground.

Calf Raises

calves (1-4)

Stand on one leg on the edge of any stair or other stable platform—a coffee table, bathtub rim, bottom rung of a ladder, even a thick phone book will do the trick—so that only the ball of your foot is on the platform and your heel's in the air. Grab hold of a banister or wall *lightly* for balance.

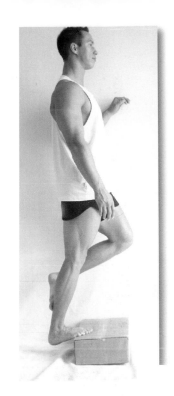

Keeping your knee only slightly bent throughout the movement, lower yourself down as far as your calf will stretch, holding it there for a second before pushing yourself up as high as possible onto the ball of your foot. Hold this peak position as well for one second.

When you can no longer get one good rep with a full range of motion, do ten quick partial reps. Then switch feet.

To focus on the insides of your calves, turn your toes slightly outward during this exercise. Similarly, to emphasize the outside of your calves, turn your toes slightly inward.

If you want to build your upper calves (*gastrocnemius*)—nice for women who want shapely calves but not thick ankles—concentrate your partial reps on the upper half of the movement (starting with your heel level with your toes and going up as high as possible). Likewise if you want to focus on your lower calves (*soleus*), which produces greater overall thickness in your calves (because the soleus wraps under the upper calves as well as going down to the ankles), execute your partial reps in the lower portion of the movement (starting at the bottom in a full stretch and pushing up as high as you can).

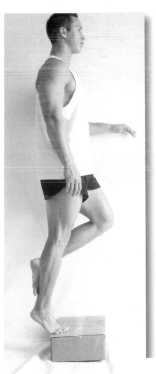

Variation: If it's too tough at first to do this with one foot at a time, try it with both feet at once.

> **Want a great calf workout?** Start at the bottom of a staircase and do one set with each foot on that bottom step, then move up to the next step. Do another set, then climb another step. Go up ten stairs without stopping and you're done with calves for the week. You should feel it the next day as your calves start blasting into shape.

You can also do "Donkey Calf Raises," a great twist to this exercise when your muscles get overly accustomed to regular Calf Raises and stop responding as much as they used to. Simply bend over at the hips about 90 degrees, holding onto something lightly for balance like a chair, a banister, or a stair a few steps up.

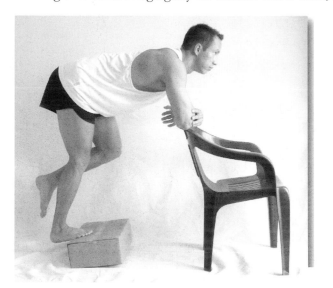 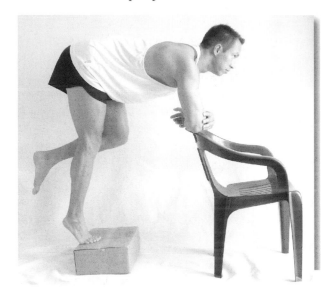

Variation: You can really strengthen your lower calves by bending at the knees throughout the movement. Just bend your knee as much as possible—typically your thigh will be at slightly less than a 90-degree angle with your shin—and stick your butt back and your shoulders forward, lightly balancing with your hands in front of you on a higher stair or something. But be sure to keep your knees bent at the exact same angle the whole time—you're not working your thighs here.

Ready to kick it up a notch? Load up a backpack with books, sand, rocks or—if you're doing Donkey Calf Raises—you can even have someone straddle your hips. I personally have an old backpack I keep filled with rocks and an old five gallon bucket always filled with water with a secure top. Holding the bucket while wearing the backpack not only really blasts my calves, but strengthens my forearms, shoulders, and traps at the same time. Typically, I'll start on my left foot, cranking out a set of standard Calf Raises holding the bucket and wearing the backpack. Then I'll put the bucket down, lean down and bend my knee, and do another ten reps of Donkey Calf Raises to hit my lower calves. Lastly, I'll stand without the bucket and finish with another ten reps of standard Calf Raises. Then I grab the bucket again, switch feet, and repeat. Then it's on up to the next stair! I'll go seven steps, and after that, all that's left to do is stick a fork in my calves, because they're done.

Another great calf workout is to do four sets of five minute Tabatas. I wear a loaded backpack and start on my left foot, doing 20 second sets of Donkey Calf Raises with my knees bent, with 10 seconds of rest in between. After five minutes, I switch to my right foot and do the same thing. Then I go back to my left foot, this time standing up straight to focus on my upper calf, still wearing the backpack. Again, I do five minutes of Tabatas (20 seconds on, 10 seconds off), then switch feet. It takes only 20 minutes, but you've done 20 sets on each leg!

The Cliffhanger
calves (4)

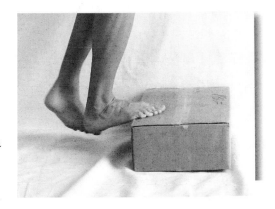

This one's all about balance and strength. Just stand on one foot on the edge of a stair or any stable platform (a bathtub rim or bottom rung of a ladder is perfect). Only the ball of your foot and your toes should be touching the surface, as if you were doing a standard one-legged Calf Raise. Here's the catch: You cannot hold onto anything. Holding your foot still, balance there as long as you can! You'll feel every last shred of calf muscle firing, and the more you struggle to balance the harder it is. Obviously, don't put yourself in danger. Always have something (a wall, a secure shower curtain rod) to grab if you lose your balance. Time yourself. When I got up to five minutes, I added a weighted back pack (about 55 pounds), and now I do it for three minutes on each foot. This is also a superb way to finish off any calf workout.

Pogo Jump
calves (2)

Keeping your knees almost straight but without your kneecaps locked, repeatedly jump as high as possible as quickly as you can without allowing your heels to touch the ground. This is a good warm-up for more advanced athletes and a good exercise for beginners to develop power in their calves.

Hop Around
calves (3)

Stand on one leg with your knee only slightly bent. Jump into the air explosively by only bending your ankle. Do this rapidly until you can no longer make it off the ground, then switch feet. Be sure to focus on pushing up off only the ball of your foot, and do not bend or straighten your knee at all.

Little Piggies
front of the calves (1-4)

Perhaps the most commonly neglected muscle group, this is a crucial area both for balance as well as to fill out your calves.

With your feet a few inches apart, place only your heels on the edge of a stair or other platform—such as a large book, coffee table, or filled box—so that the rest of your feet hang off. Hold onto something like a wall or banister *lightly* for balance. Keeping your knees in a fixed, slightly bent position, point your toes as far down as possible, then simply raise them as high as possible. All your weight should be on your heels, and nothing but your feet should move. Repeat until you can't do another full rep.

Because of the limited range of movement (as with all calf exercises), for the best workout, you should keep doing as many partial reps as well as you can for thirty seconds after you can't do another full rep.

Ready to kick it up a notch? Let go. Put your hands out for balance but don't hold onto anything at all. This dramatically increases the efficacy of this exercise.

When you can do thirty Little Piggies without holding onto anything, then try starting with one foot at a time (you'll need to hold onto something lightly), then the next foot, and after you've exhausted both calves, do them together without holding onto anything.

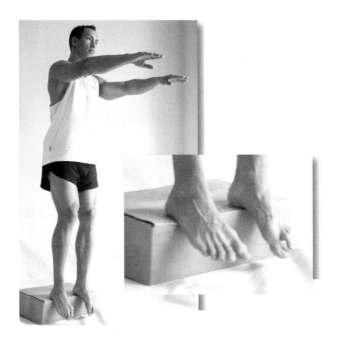 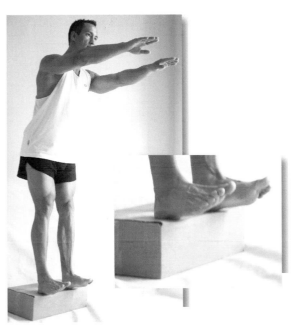

CORE Exercises

Your core is just that: the center of your entire body. It's importance in form, function and fashion cannot be overestimated. 90% of backaches can be eliminated by strengthening your core muscles. In addition to making pain history, a strong core will let you look great on the beach now and carry your grandkids around in the future—instead of having them carry you around in a wheelchair. This section runs the gamut from how to do the most effective Crunches and Supermans to Hello Darlings and Russian Twists to elite exercises like Jack Knives and Flags, and finishes up with exercises to strengthen your neck.

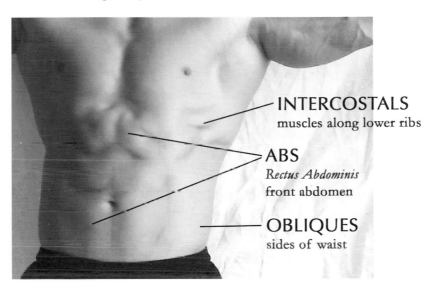

INTERCOSTALS
muscles along lower ribs

ABS
Rectus Abdominis
front abdomen

OBLIQUES
sides of waist

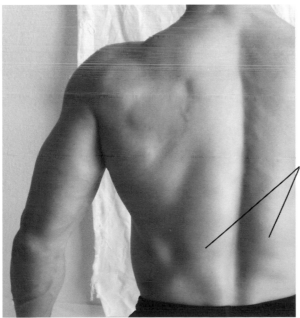

ERECTOR SPINAE
muscles surrounding
the lumbar region of
the lower back

Standing Knee Raises

abs (1)

Stand upright, feet slightly apart, then raise your left knee as high as possible. Hold it up for three seconds. Balancing like this will also help develop all your leg muscles in your standing leg. Then lower your leg slowly, and raise your right knee in the same manner.

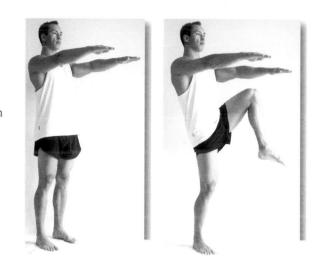

Beach Scissors

hip flexors, obliques (1-3)

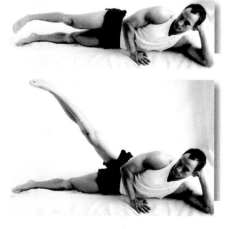

Lying on your left side with your left hand propping your head up, raise your right leg as high as possible, keeping it straight. Hold for three seconds. Return to starting position and repeat. When you're finished, just flip over and do the same on the other side.

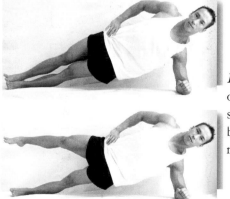

Ready to kick it up a notch? Do this exercise while propping yourself up on your elbow. Your whole body, from your head down to your bottom foot, should remain in a straight line. This is superior to standard Beach Scissors because it strengthens all your core muscles, especially the sides of your abdomen.

Russian Twists

abs, intercostals, obliques (1)

Sit upright on the ground with your arms crossed and knees bent. Lift your feet off the ground. Twist so that your left elbow touches your right knee, then twist the other way so that your right elbow touches your left knee. Go back and forth, twisting as much as you can at the waist, without lowering your legs. If you like, you can cross your ankles.

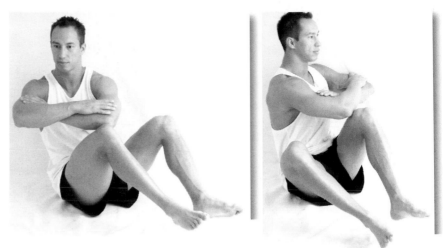

Hip Ups

tones every muscle from shoulders to ankles, with special emphasis on your obliques and intercostals (3)

Lie on your right side with your right elbow directly underneath your shoulder. Place your left foot on top of your right foot. Now, raise your pelvis off the ground so that your body's straight from head to heels and your pelvis is forward and in line with the rest of your body. Slowly lower your hip back to the ground. Do ten reps then switch sides.

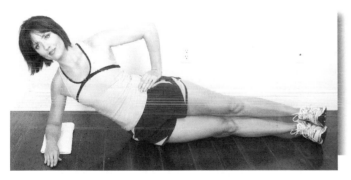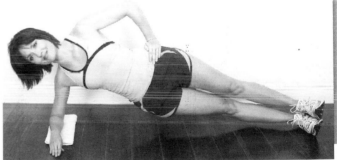

Variation: If this is too difficult, try getting up on your knees rather than your feet. You'll have to bend your knees slightly to get your lower legs out of the way.

You can also support yourself on one hand with your arm straight, rather than on an elbow, which makes it a little more difficult.

Ready to kick it up a notch? Hold yourself up for as long as you can. Try for a whole minute. Once you can do that, try holding the top leg up in the air. Another great way to crank this one up a notch and really develop some great obliques is to lightly pump your hips up and down, in the top portion of the movement, for as long as possible.

Crunch It Ups

abs, with particular focus on the upper abs (1 - 2)

A favorite of some Marines I used to train with. Lie flat on your back. With your knees bent (the closer your butt is to your feet, the easier this exercise is), tuck your feet under something (bed, couch, chair, bookcase, coffee table, etc.). Cross your arms in front of your stomach. Keeping your arms pressed against your stomach, bring your upper body up just enough to touch your elbows to the very bottoms of your thighs then go back down until your shoulder blades touch the ground again. There is very little range of motion in this exercise, and yet it's greatly effective.

Try doing 100 of these, no matter how many sets it takes you. As your abs get more and more developed, it'll take you less and less sets, until someday you can crank out 100 straight and your abs are hard as a rock.

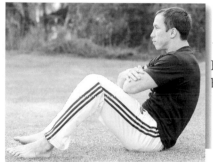

Variation: You can increase the difficulty by increasing the range of motion. Don't hook your feet under anything and bring your elbows out away from your body so they touch your thighs closer to your knees.

Crunches

upper abs (1)

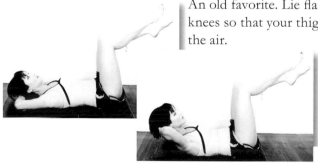

An old favorite. Lie flat on your back. Put your hands under your head, bend your knees so that your thighs are perpendicular to the ground, and cross your ankles in the air.

Pull your chest toward your knees. As with all these exercises, keep your chin about a fist's length from your chest to avoid placing unnecessary strain on your neck. Hold at the top for a moment while you exhale powerfully. Then come back down. Your range of motion should be quite small, maybe only moving your shoulders a few inches off the ground.

Variations: These are especially effective if you can do them without letting your shoulder blades ever touch the ground.

You can also do Side Crunches by crunching forward and twisting to the side so that your left elbow touches your right kneecap, then immediately bring your right elbow to your left knee, then lower your shoulders and repeat. Or bring your left elbow to your right knee, then lower your shoulders, then bring your right elbow to your left knee… back and forth… you get the idea.

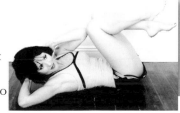

Leg Lifts

lower abs, hip flexors (1-2)

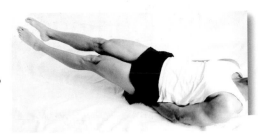

Lie down on your back with your hands under your butt and your head up (this will help strengthen your neck).

Start with your legs straight, together, and six inches off the ground, and then lift your feet up until your legs are at a 45-degree angle with the ground. Be sure to keep your knees straight. Hold for 2 seconds, then return your legs to the ground slowly and repeat the movement.

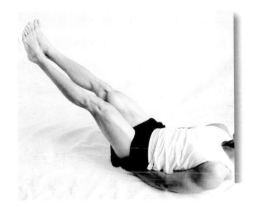

Variation: Start with your legs at a 45-degree angle to the ground and bring them up until they are at a 90-degree angle.

To increase the difficulty, place your hands on your chest.

Ready to kick it up a notch? Want to have some fun? Write your whole name in the air with your feet together and legs straight, one letter at a time. I learned this one from the Ukrainian military.

Flutter Kicks

lower abs, hip flexors (2)

Lie down on your back with your hands under your butt and your head up. Keeping your legs straight and together, lift your feet into the air, six-inches from the ground.

Keeping it straight, raise your right leg up to three feet in the air, and then bring it back down even with your left leg which is still six inches above the ground. Repeat the movement with your left leg. This can be done swiftly or slowly. Just be sure to keep the motion very controlled.

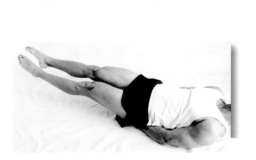
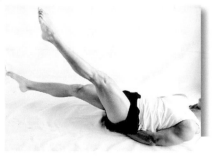
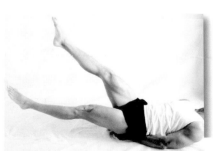

Variation: Place your hands on your chest to make it a bit harder.

Hello Darlings

lower abs, hip flexors (2)

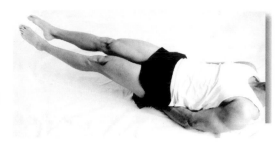

Lie down on your back with your hands under your butt and your head up (this helps strengthen your neck). Keeping your legs straight, lift your feet into the air, about six inches above the ground. Open your legs as wide as possible, then close them.

Ready to kick it up a notch? Place your hands on your chest to increase the difficulty of this one.

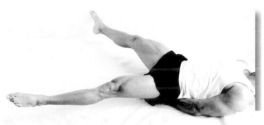

You can also cross your ankles at the end of each rep, rather than merely bringing your feet together. Change which foot is on top after each rep.

Bicycles

one of the best for overall development of the abs, intercostals and obliques (2)

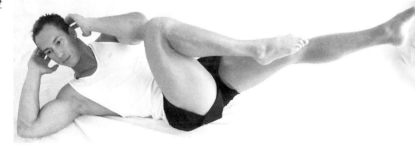

Lie down on your back with your legs straight and you hands under your head. Hold one leg up, fully extended, about six inches off the ground. Pull the knee of your other leg in toward your chest, and touch it with your opposite elbow. Now begin "bicycling" and touch each knee with the opposite elbow as it comes in toward your chest. Be sure to extend each leg fully before bringing it back in to your chest.

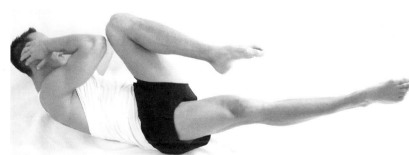

The key to making these really effective is to do them slow and controlled. Doing 10 very slow repetitions will strengthen your mid-region more than doing 30 of them fast.

V-Ups

abs, hip flexors (2)

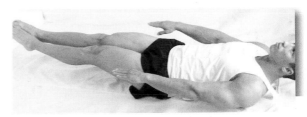

One of the greatest exercises for your abs.

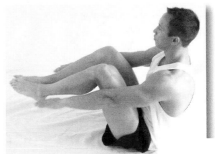

Lie flat on your back, arms to your side. Keeping only your butt on the ground, bring your chest and your knees up toward each other, almost until they touch. Then lean your chest back and straighten your legs out so that both your shoulders and feet are each just a few inches off the ground.

Variation: Know as "Rowers," you can use your hands like you're rowing a boat, extending your arms straight out as you bring your knees in, and then bringing your hands into your chest as you extend your legs and lean back. Be sure to bend only at the elbows, and keep your elbows fixed in the same place out from your body.

Side V-Ups

intercostals, obliques, abs (3)

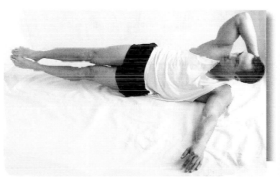
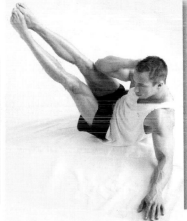

Lie on your left side with your left arm sticking out straight in front of you on the floor, palm down. Place your right hand on your head, with your elbow sticking up toward the ceiling. Keeping your legs together and straight, and bending only at the hips, bring your knees to your right elbow. Your legs should now be at a 90-degree angle to your upper body. Lower your legs back to the ground slowly, without letting your feet touch the ground before your next rep.

Iron Crosses

abs, obliques, intercostals (3)

Lie on your back with your legs pointing straight up into the air, so that they are at a 90-degree angle with your upper body. Put your arms straight out on the floor, perpendicular to your body, with palms down on the floor. With your head off the ground, lower your legs to the right, so that your body is still in an L shape. Just before your legs touch the ground, raise them back up to the upright position and lower them to the opposite side.

Variation: Doing this exercise with your knees bent makes it easier.

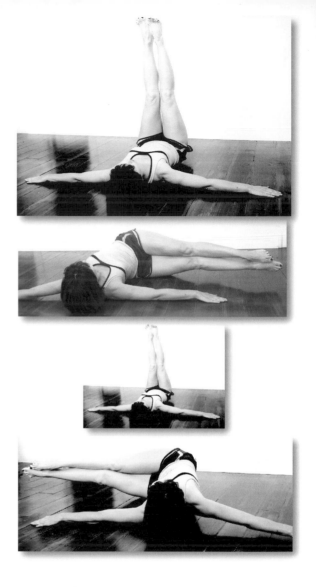

Jack Knives

abs, hip flexors (3)

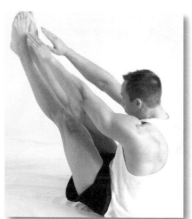

This one's only for those with some real strong abs and coordination.

Lie flat on your back, with your feet six inches off the ground and your arms extended straight up over your head. Keeping only your butt on the ground, simultaneously bring your chest up and your straight legs up until your hands touch your feet. Then lean your chest and arms back and bring your legs down until both your shoulders and feet are just a few inches off the ground.

Variation: To make this a little easier, you can bring your shoulders all the way back down to the ground at the bottom of the movement.

YOU ARE YOUR OWN GYM

Hanging Leg Lifts

abs, hip flexors, forearms (3-4)

Find something to hold onto and hang your entire body from it. It's best if it's high enough that your feet are off the ground when hanging. But if you can't find or reach something that high, it's okay to use something only high enough that your feet are on the floor and your legs are somewhat bent. I've used door frames, door tops, Pull Up bars, tree limbs, the edge of a porch, and the top of a swing set like in this photo. While hanging, bring your knees up toward your chest. Then let them back down without swinging.

Variation: Bringing your legs to your sides, one after the other, will place more emphasis on the muscles along your ribs and beneath your ribs (intercostals and obliques).

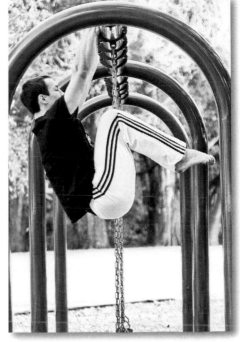

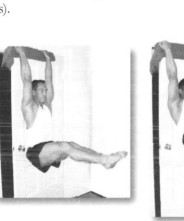

Ready to kick it up a notch? Once you've mastered the bent leg lifts, try doing this exercise with your legs straight! For the elite, I suggest bringing your feet all the way up to your hands (or as close as your flexibility will allow) and back down without swinging. You'll have to be incredibly flexible and strong to do this on a door, while it's easier using something that does not block your upper body from moving back a little during the top of the movement, like a Pull Up bar.

Flags

abs, obliques, with a minor focus on your triceps and forearms (4)

This one is only for the elite!

Lie flat on your back and hook your hands under something that is close to the top of your head and fixed to the ground (or at least very heavy, like a couch with someone sitting on it). Keeping your entire body dead straight (except your neck), raise your whole body into the air so that only your shoulders and head are touching the ground. Hold for two seconds, then let your body fall slowly, in a controlled manner, back to the ground.

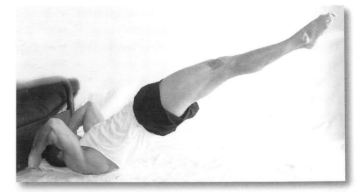

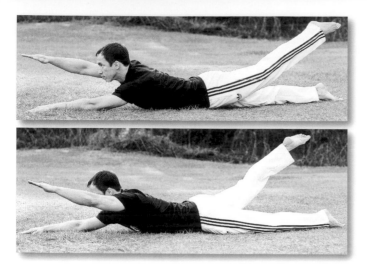

Swimmers

glutes, lower back (2)

Lie down flat on your stomach with your arms straight out in front of you. Lift only your right leg and your left arm, as high as possible. Hold for three seconds, then lower them slowly. Then raise your left leg and right arm. Again, hold for three seconds, and lower them. Switch back and forth.

Supermans

glutes, lower back (3)

Lie down flat on your stomach with your arms out straight in front of you. Keeping your legs and arms straight, lift them all off the ground as high as possible, so that only your torso and pelvis are still on the ground. Hold this for a three seconds and repeat.

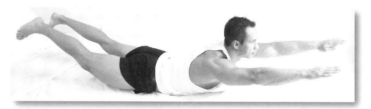

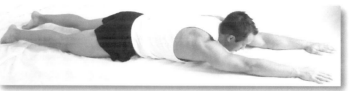

Variations: There are several different alternative # Hyperextensions that work similar muscles. You can place your hands along the side of your body, or under your chin and raise them up at the same time as your legs, just like Supermans. A favorite of mine is what I call "The Flying Jesus," where you hold your arms straight out to your sides so that they are at 90-degree angles with your body.

Pillow Humpers

glutes, lower back, hamstrings, spinal erectors, back of neck (3)

Lie on your stomach with your feet hooked under something like a couch, or if you don't have anything, put them flat against a wall, using the friction between your feet and the wall to keep your legs stationary. Place a tightly rolled up pillow underneath your hips. With your hands behind your head, lift your upper body off the ground as high as possible while keeping your toes on the ground. Look up toward the ceiling at the top of the movement and really squeeze your back muscles and glutes tight.

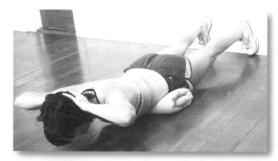

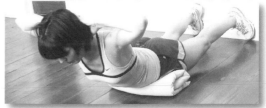

YOU ARE YOUR OWN GYM

Core Stabilization

strengthens almost every muscle in your body from your shoulders to your calves, especially your entire core—abs, lower back, glutes, hip flexors (2)

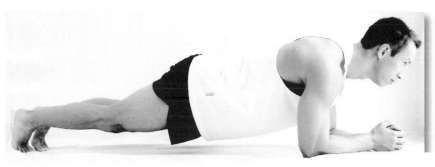

As simple as it is effective. Lie down on your stomach then prop yourself up on your elbows, bent at 90 degrees, shoulder-width apart, so that your forearms are on the ground. You may want to place your elbows on a pillow for comfort. Hold this position for as long as you can. One to two minutes is great. Be sure to keep your pelvis down and your body straight from head to heels. Rest 30 seconds. Repeat.

Variation: Static Push Ups. Simply freeze in the starting position of a Push Up, holding your arms locked straight out. In addition to working your core, this will strengthen your shoulders, triceps, and pectorals.

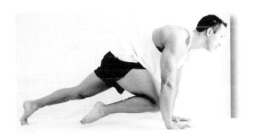

Once you can handle this, try doing the same exercise, only this time bring your right knee up toward your chest. Hold it there for 3 seconds, then return it to the ground, and pull in your left knee.

Ready to kick it up a notch? Try holding a static Push Up with your arms bent at 90 degrees.

S&M Push Ups

all core muscles as well as pectorals, triceps, and deltoids (1-3)

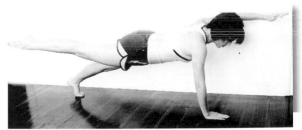

Start in the Classic Push Up position, then lift one leg straight up behind you, and extend your opposite arm straight out in front of you. Keep your head up and make yourself as long as possible. Hold as long as you can before switching to the other arm and other leg.

Variation: To make this movement easier start from the crawling position—hands and knees on the ground—and keep one knee on the ground throughout the exercise. To make this a lot more difficult, perform a One-Arm Push Up while holding one arm and the opposite leg fully extended.

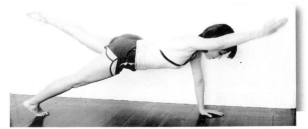

Yes, No, Maybe's

neck (1-4)

This is a great way to alleviate current neck problems and fend off future ones. The neck contains typically completely overlooked muscles. Don't be that guy who's worked hard to develop big shoulders, pecs and traps, only to have a little pencil neck shooting out of your collar.

Lie on your back on a table, desk or bed with your head hanging off the edge. Move your head straight up and down as though you're nodding ("Yes's").

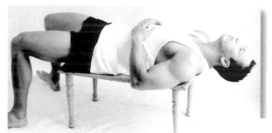
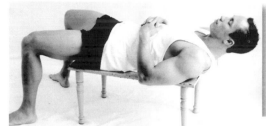

Or move your head side to side bringing each ear near to its corresponding shoulder, with a pause in the middle ("Maybe's").

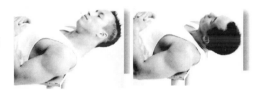

Or turn your head so that you are looking to the right and then turn to the left, pausing in the middle ("No's").

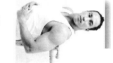

Yet another great one is rolling your head around in slow circles, switching direction every other set.

To work the back of your neck, lie belly down (or kneel with your head hanging forward) and move your head up and down with your hands interlaced behind your head, trying to pull your head downward.

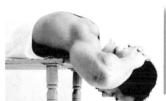
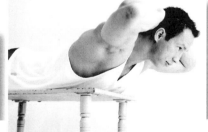

Ready to kick it up a notch? Put the back of either wrist on your forehead while holding onto the opposite wrist, and try to push your head down toward the ground for added resistance on Yes's or Maybe's.

Once your neck is strong enough, you can also hold any kind of weight on your forehead, and do any of the above exercises. A dictionary, telephone book, or even a good-sized rock or cinder block with a towel folded under it will do the trick.

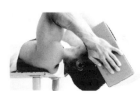
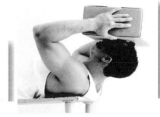

EXTRA, EXTRA:

Some great all around butt kickers!

Some of these compound movements may seem a little tough to get the hang of at first, but they're actually quite simple and well worth the effort. I don't know how many workouts I've done at the end of a long day, or in a time crunch, consisting entirely of 100 8-Count Bodybuilders in a row. It's tough, that's for sure, but it takes less than 10 minutes and you'll have one heck of a workout. If that seems like too much for now, try just doing 50 4-Count Bodybuilders, no matter how many sets it takes you. When you can finally do 50 straight, without resting, try 55, then 60, until you reach 100. Start with 4-Count Bodybuilders and work up to Burpees and 8-Count Bodybuilders. Just remember: if you're only going to do one set, you better put out!

4-Count Bodybuilders

pectorals, triceps, shoulders, core, lats, hip flexors (3)

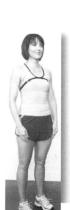

Stand erect, feet together. Squat down and put your hands on the ground, just out-side of your feet (Count 1).

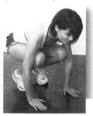

Kick your feet out so that you are in Push Up starting position (2).

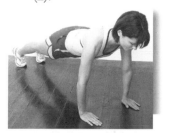

Jump your feet back up so that your knees are again at your chest and you're in a deep Squat (3).

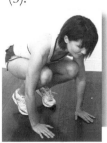

Stand up (4).

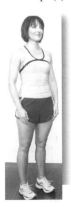

Burpees

pectorals, triceps, shoulders, core, lats, hip flexors, quadriceps, glutes, calves (3)

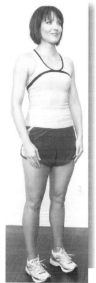

Stand with your feet together. Place your hands on the ground in front of your feet.

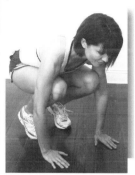

Kick both feet out so that you land in the Classic Push Up starting position.

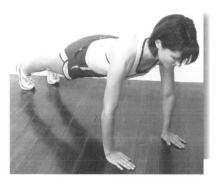

Perform a Push Up.

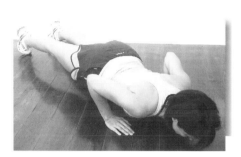

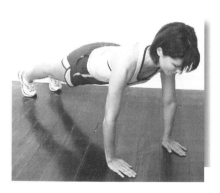

Jump your feet back up toward your chest, and land in the squatting position.

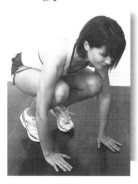

Jump into the air with your arms overhead

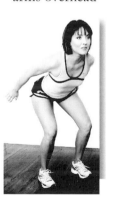

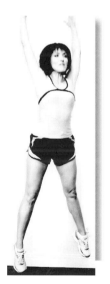

Land and repeat the movement.

Variation: If doing a Push Up on the ground is still a bit tough, try doing this exercise with your hands elevated on something like a coffee table or the edge of a couch.

8-Count Bodybuilders

pectorals, triceps, shoulders, core, lats, hip flexors (3)

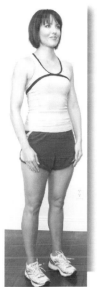

Stand with your feet together. Place your hands on the ground in front of your feet (count 1).

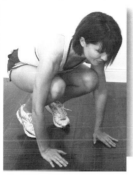

Kick both feet out so that you land in the Classic Push Up starting position (2).

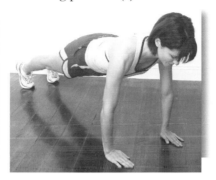

Perform a Push Up (3).

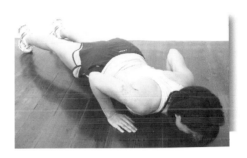

(And 4.)

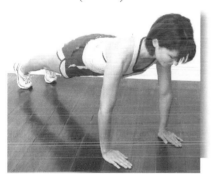

Kick your feet apart (5).

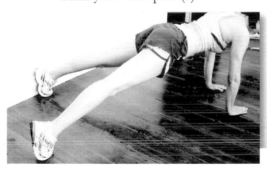

Bring them together (6).

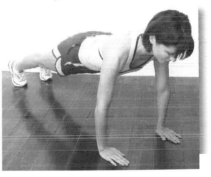

Bring both feet, simultaneously, to your hands (7).

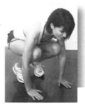

Stand-up (8!).

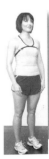

Ready to kick it up a notch? Try kicking your feet apart while in the bottom of the Push Up position to make this exercise harder. The tighter and more perfect your form is, the harder and more productive this exercise becomes.

Spidermans (4)

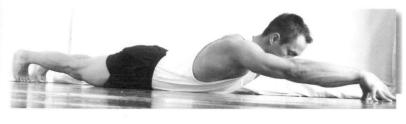

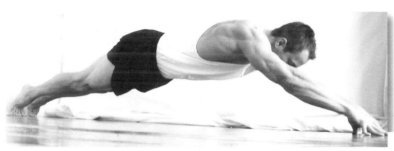

This elite exercise works pretty much your whole body, with special emphasis on your core, back and chest. You should be thoroughly warmed-up before executing this movement.

Lay flat on your stomach with your arms stretched out ahead of you. Bend your wrists, place your fingertips on the ground, and place the balls of your feet on the ground. Now, take a deep breath, hold it, tighten your abdomen, tuck your pubic bone, and drive your midsection up off the ground. This one's no joke! In order to protect your lower back, make sure your midsection is rock hard while performing this exercise.

Variation: Perform the exercise exactly the same, but instead of placing your hands in front of you, place them out to the sides. This will put more emphasis on your pecs, and make the exercise a bit easier.

You can also place your palms down on the floor, thus taking the strain off your fingers.

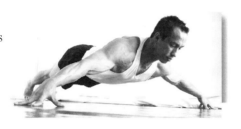

Ready to kick it up a notch? Start with your belly on the floor, but your hands and feet up on low surfaces, like telephone books.

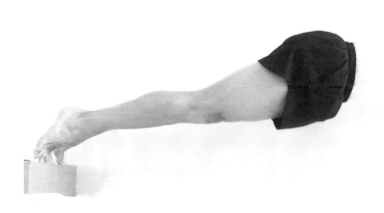

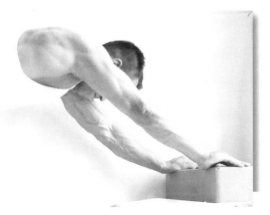

Farmer's Walk

works virtually every muscle in your body (4)

Simply grab the heaviest things you can hold in each hand (or one thing in both hands) and start walking until you have to drop them. Keep your back straight, and your midsection rock-solid tight. Get creative here. Use water cooler jugs, cinder blocks tied or chained together, bags or backpacks full of sand or rocks, whatever you can think of. Go to the junk yard and see what you can find—an old refrigerator, an engine, car parts, anything.

Horse Power

every muscle in your body (4)

Put your car in neutral on a flat, unused road or driveway. Make sure it does not coast in any direction. Then push it as far as you can! Who knows, someday you could be on ESPN competing in the World's Strongest Man competition.

Send me pics of yourself trying some of these out at MarkLauren.com.

12.   THE PROGRAM

THIS IS FOR THOSE WHO WOULD RATHER follow a simple, specific program than construct their own. Exercise just 4 or 5 times a week for 20 - 30 minutes, for 10-week cycles.

Unlike weight-training programs, not everyone can do the same exercises and simply shift the size of the dumbbell they lift. Different ability levels dictate different exercises, but the workout programs for the Basic (beginner), 1st class (intermediate), Master (advanced), and Chief (elite) levels are all based off the same sound training principles, and various types of "periodization." More about periodization and the science behind the program, if you're interested, can be found in Appendix 3.

Some beginners may see only a small difference in their overall weight, but their waists will thin while their muscle tone will increase. We're talking *body composition* here, which is far more important than simply looking at the scales to measure the validity of a fitness program.

You must be patient. If you're overweight and haven't exercised in a decade, you can't just suddenly undo 10 years of neglect in 2 months. If you stick with the program, you will eventually get your body where you want it, but to be successful in the long-term it must inherently be a slow process. As I've said, losing .5 pounds per week is optimal for a woman, a little more for a man. Don't torture yourself by checking the scales every day. This program is designed to be as effective as possible without overlooking long-term goals. It is not designed to be a two-month, one-shot, fixed-it-for-good routine. Any book, product, program, pill or diet claiming such a thing should be burned.

Over the course of ten years, I carefully designed this program to get maximal results in as little time as possible, not just for ten weeks or even ten years, but for life. When you finish one cycle, you can take a week or two off, and then get on another one, endlessly maximizing gains and, at the same time, preventing burnout. As you reach greater and greater levels of fitness, you'll only need to plug in more difficult exercises or variations. So the program outlines never change. Only the exercises themselves change.

Each 10-week program consists of four periods called **blocks**. Each block utilizes different types of workouts that are explained fully below. A quick summary:

- The **Muscular Endurance Block** (weeks 1 - 2) uses "Ladders," low on intensity but high on reps, in order to promote movement proficiency.

- In the **Strength Training Block** (weeks 3 - 4), each day you'll do four different exercises, 3 sets of 6-12 reps for each, at 3-minute intervals. We're cranking it up a notch in intensity from the first two weeks, yet there will be less reps overall.

- During the **Power Block** (weeks 5 - 6), exercises are paired together in "Supersets." The first exercise in each pair will be the more difficult one and will be done in 1 - 5 reps. Immediately after, you'll do 6 - 12 reps of another exercise. Each Superset is done at a four-minute interval.

- Finally, the **Undulating Block** (weeks 6 - 10) will employ all the methods used so far, as well as some new ones like "Stappers" and "Tabatas." No two training days in a week will use the same type of workout, and each week a different type of workout is used to train pushing movements, pulling movements, leg movements, and core movements. Here you'll add one day to your workout schedule, making it five days, but that's it, and two of the five workouts are only 16 and 20 minutes long.

Once you become more familiar with your capabilities and the exercises, you'll want to start customizing your program, deviating from the exercises that are outlined. Have fun, go wild. Again, only once you take the bull by the horns and achieve autonomy in your fitness regime will you reach your body's potential. Ultimately, *you* are the only one who knows what's best for *you*. Just be sure to follow these simple rules:

- Don't replace movements from a particular category with movements from another. For example, don't replace a leg exercise with a pushing exercise.

- Definitely don't choose exercises because they're the most comfortable! Getting into shape requires that you occasionally let go of your comfort. Don't swallow the infomercials' lies, where 22-year-old men and women are smiling without a trace of sweat while getting into amazing shape on some new fitness gadget. You're going to have to work.

- Be sure you can always do the required amount of reps with good form, while at the same time not exceeding the required amount of reps.

- Stick with mainly compound exercises, those that require the use of two or more joints, such as shoulders and elbows (Push Up) or hips and knees (Squat). They develop greater balance, increase heart rate further, stimulate more muscle growth, and are more functional than isolation exercises. (When is the last time you did anything strenuous using only one muscle?) You'll notice my program is a bit lighter on ab exercises than many other programs. No doubt about it: Athletes who practice compound movements that involve core stabilization tend to have stronger mid-sections than some guy who sits on the gym floor cranking out crunches. When choosing exercises, place the compound movements that work the biggest muscles first.

See my website <u>MarkLauren.com</u> for some even shorter, but more intense, 20-minute workouts!

Hooya!

PERIODIZATION

It's normal for our progress to have occasional dips and valleys for various reasons, so don't let it discourage you. Three steps forward, one step back; four steps forward, two steps back... That's just how it goes, as it does with most things in life. Our bodies cannot simply progress in a linear manner indefinitely. Eventually, our limited recuperative energy falls short of the demands placed on it, and you'll get stuck in a rut. The "periodization" utilized in my programs was developed to combat this. It balances periods of high-intensity with less demanding periods that focus on movement proficiency and muscular endurance.

THE WORKOUTS:

LADDERS

Perform 1 rep of any exercise, rest, perform 2 reps, rest, perform 3 reps, etc... until going any higher would cause you to hit muscle failure on subsequent sets. Once you've reached that point, come back down without repeating the highest number. The rest intervals will be the same as your previous work interval. So you'll have more rest as the numbers get higher, and less rest as the numbers get lower on the way back down to 1.

Each exercise in this block will be done with 7.5 minutes of Ladders. If you've reached the bottom of your Ladder (1 rep) and the set time (7.5 minutes) hasn't expired, simply start another ladder. Similarly, you may not even reach the bottom of your ladder, and that's okay too.

Train yourself to perform the exercises correctly. If you reach muscle failure at any point during your ladder workout, you went too high before coming back down. This is meant to be a high-volume/low-intensity workout.

It is okay to perform the ladder workout in the low rep range—possibly even repeating single reps towards the end of the workout, in order to avoid hitting failure.

Exercises where you alternate sides are done by performing the designated number of reps on both sides before resting.

INTERVAL SETS

- Three sets per exercise.
- 6 - 12 reps per set.
- 3-minute intervals. Start time when beginning an exercise, go to failure or up to 1.5 minutes, and rest for the remainder of the interval.
- For all single limb movements, like Bulgarian Split Squats, One-Legged Romanian Dead Lifts (RDLs), and Side Lunges, do one side at a time. Start with the non-dominant side and immediately switch to the dominant side.

SUPERSETS

- 4 minute intervals for each set.
- Perform 1 - 5 reps for the first set, and 6 - 12 reps for the exercise that immediately follows.
- 2 sets per exercise pair.
- The first exercise in each pair should *not* be done to failure.
- Perform all movements with as much control as possible! The first exercise in each pair should be done with slow negative movements (2 - 3 seconds) and controlled, explosive concentric movements (about 1 second) with a 1 second pause at the beginning and end of each movement.
- For single limb exercises, alternate sides after each rep.

STAPPERS

Repeat as many cycles of the given exercises and repetitions as possible in 20 minutes, with no rest in between. If you have to take short breaks because of muscle failure, it's okay, but try to keep rest to a minimum.

TABATAS

8 rounds of 20 seconds of exercise followed by 10 seconds of rest, for a total of 4 minutes. This is high-intensity training. Exercises done for Tabatas should be executed as fast as possible. Keep rest time to a minimum if failure is reached during a 20-second work period.

If you want to keep track of your reps for each exercise each day, you can download log sheets at MarkLauren.com.

Basic Program

for Beginners

~Weeks 1 & 2~

Muscular Endurance Block
(Ladders)

	Day 1 Push/Pull	Day 2 Legs/Core	Day 3 Push/Pull	Day 4 Legs/Core
Exercises:	Push Ups w/hands elevated on platform	Alternating Back Lunges	Push Ups w/hands elevated on platform	Side Lunges
	Let Me Ins	Alternating 1-Legged RDLs*	Let Me Ins	Alternating 1-Legged RDLs
	Seated Dips w/ feet on ground	Squats	Seated Dips w/ feet on ground	Squats w/1-3 second pause at bottom
	Let Me Ups w/knees bent	Swimmers	Let Me Ups w/knees bent	Side Crunches

*Romanian Dead Lifts

~Weeks 3 & 4~

Strength Block
(Interval Sets)

	Day 1/ Push	Day 2/ Legs	Day 3/ Pull	Day 4/ Core
Exercises:	Push Ups	Bulgarian Split Squats	Let Me Ins	Leg Lifts
	Military Press w/hands elevated	Side Lunges	Let Me Ups w/knees bent	Hyperextensions w/hands under chin
	Close Grip Push Ups w/hands elevated	Squats w/1-3 second pause at bottom	Let Me Ins w/ palms up	Russian Twists
	Seated Dips	1-Legged RDLs on pillow	Towel Curls	Swimmers

~Weeks 5 & 6~

Power Block
(Supersets)

	Day 1/ Push	Day 2/ Legs	Day 3/ Pull	Day 4/ Core
Exercises:	Push Ups w/feet elevated & Shove Offs	Alternating Back Lunges w/4-6 second pause at bottom & Toyotas	Assisted Door Pull Ups (use a chair to place your feet on or jump and concentrate on the negative) & Let Me Ins	V-Ups & Russian Twists
	Military Press & Thumbs Up	Alternating Front Lunges w/4-6 second pause at bottom & Side Lunges	Let Me Ins w/ 4-6 second contraction at top & Towel Curls	Supermans & Swimmers
	Close Grip Push Ups & Seated Dips	Alternating 1-Legged RDLs on pillow & Squats w/1-3 second pause at bottom	Let Me Ups w/reverse grip and straight legs & Let Me Ins w/palms up	Hanging Leg Lifts w/knees bent & Leg Lifts

~Weeks 7-10~

Undulating Block

	Day 1/ Push	Day 2/ Leg	Day 3/ Pull	Day 4/ Core	Day 5
Week 7	**Ladders** Military Press w/hands elevated, Push Ups w/hands elevated, Close Grip Push Ups w/hands elevated, Seated Dips w/ knees bent	**Super Sets** Alternating Back Lunges w/4-6 second pause at bottom & Toyotas, Alternating Front Lunges w/4-6 second pause at bottom & Side Lunges, Alternating1-Legged RDLs on pillow and 1-3 second pause at middle & Pogo Jumps	**Interval Sets** Let Me Ins, Let Me Ups w/knees bent, Let Me Ins w/ palms up, Towel Curls	**Tabatas** Russian Twists, Beach Scissors, Standing Knee Raises	**Stappers** 10 Alternating Back Lunges, 8 Let Me Ins, 6 Push Ups

Week 8	**Tabatas** Push Ups w/ hands elevated about chest high, Rocking Chairs, Burpees w/ hands elevated about waist high	**Ladders** Alternating Back Lunges, Alternating 1-Legged RDLs, Squats w/ 1-3 second pause at bottom, Good Mornings w/1-3 second pause at bottom	**Super Sets** Assisted Door Pull Ups (use a chair to place your feet on or jump and concentrate on the negative) & Let Me Ins, Let Me Ins w/4-6 second contraction at top & Let Me Ups w/knees bent, Let Me Ups w/reverse grip and straight legs & Let Me Ins w/palms up	**Interval Sets** Leg Lifts, Hyperextensions w/hands under chin, Russian Twists, Swimmers	**Stappers** 10 Alternating Back Lunges, 8 Let Me Ins, 6 Push Ups
Week 9	**Interval Sets** Push Ups, Military Press w/hands elevated, Close Grip Push Ups w/ hands elevated	**Tabatas** Beat Your Boots, Lunges, Good Mornings	**Ladders** Let Me Ups w/knees bent, Let Me Ins, Let Me Ups w/reverse grip and knees bent, Let Me Ins w/palms up	**Super Sets** V-Ups & Russian Twists, Supermans & Swimmers, Bicycles & Leg Lifts	**Stappers** 10 Alternating Back Lunges, 8 Let Me Ins, 6 Push Ups

Week 10	Super Sets	Interval Sets	Tabatas	Ladders	Stappers
	Push Ups w/feet elevated & Shove Offs, Military Press & Thumbs Up, Close Grip Push Ups & Seated Dips w/feet on ground	Bulgarian Split Squats, Side Lunges, Squat w/ 4-6 second pause at bottom, 1-Legged RDLs on pillow	Let Me Ins w/feet behind hands (take a step back from where your feet normally are), Bam Bams, Towel Curls	Crunch It Ups, Hyperextensions w/arms at side, Leg Lifts, Hyperextensions w/lower body only	10 Alternating Back Lunges, 8 Let Me Ins, 6 Push Ups

1st Class Program

for Intermediate Level trainees

~Weeks 1 & 2~

Muscular Endurance Block
(Ladders)

	Day 1 Push/Pull	Day 2 Legs/Core	Day 3 Push/Pull	Day 4 Legs/Core
Exercises:	Push Ups	Alternating Back Lunges w/ 1-3 second pause at bottom	Push Ups	Alternating Side Lunges w/ 1-3 second pause at bottom
	Let Me Ups	Alternating 1-Legged RDLs	Let Me Ups	Alternating 1-Legged RDLs
	Military Press	Toyotas w/1-3 second pause at bottom	Military Press	Toyotas w/1-3 second pause at bottom
	Let Me Ins	Hyperextensions w/arms at side	Let Me Ins	Russian Twists

~Weeks 3 & 4~

Strength Block
(Interval Sets)

	Day 1/ Push	Day 2/ Legs	Day 3/ Pull	Day 4/ Core
Exercises:	Push Ups w/feet elevated	Bulgarian Split Squat w/1-3 second pause at bottom	Assisted Door Pull Ups (use a chair to place your feet on or jump and concentrate on the negative)	Leg Lifts w/hands on chest
	Military Press	Side Lunges w/ 4-6 second pause at bottom	Let Me Ups	Supermans
	Close Grip Push Ups	Toyotas w/4-6 second pause at bottom	Let Me Ins	Bicycles
	Assisted Dips (legs bent behind you and feet on a chair to help push up)	1-Legged RDLs on pillow	Towel Curls	Hyperextensions w/hands under chin

~Weeks 5 & 6~

Power Block
(Supersets)

	Day 1/ Push	Day 2/ Legs	Day 3/ Pull	Day 4/ Core
Exercises:	Push Ups w/feet elevated and 1-3 second pause at bottom & Shove Offs	Alternating 1-Legged Squats while holding onto chairs with both hands & Toyotas w/4-6 second pause at bottom	Door Pull Ups & Let Me Ins	Hanging Leg Lifts w/knees bent & Iron Crosses w/knees bent
	Military Press w/feet elevated & Thumbs Up	Alternating Side Lunges w/4-6 second pause at bottom & Alternating Back Lunges w/1-3 second pauses at bottom	Let Me Ins w/4-6 second contraction at top & Let Me Ups	Alternating 1-Legged Hip Extensions & Supermans
	Close Grip Push Ups w/feet elevated & Assisted Dips	Alternating 1-Legged RDLs on pillow and 1-3 second pause at bottom & Box Jumps	Let Me Ups w/reverse grip and feet elevated & Let Me Ins w/palms up	V-Ups & Russian Twists

The Program   151

~Weeks 7-10~

Undulating Block

	Day 1/ Push	Day 2/ Leg	Day 3/ Pull	Day 4/ Core	Day 5
Week 7	Ladders Chinese Push Ups, Push Ups, Close Grip Push Ups, Seated Dips	Super Sets Alternating 1-Legged Squats while holding onto two chairs & Toyotas w/4-6 second pause at bottom, Alternating Side Lunges w/4-6 second pause at bottom & Alternating Back Lunges w/1-3 second pause, Alternating 1-Legged RDLs on pillow and 1-3 second pause & Box Jumps	Interval Sets Assisted Door Pull Ups (use a chair to place your feet on or jump and concentrate on the negative), Let Me Ups, Let Me Ins, Towel Curls	Tabatas Russian Twists, Flutter Kicks, Squats	Stappers 6 Let Me Ups w/knees bent, 12 Alternating Side Lunges, 8 Push Ups

Week 8	**Tabatas** Push Ups w/hands elevated on platform, Seated Dips w/feet on ground, Squats	**Ladders** Alternating Back Lunges w/1-3 second pause at bottom, Alternating Side Lunges, Toyotas w/1-3 seconds at bottom Alternating 1-Legged RDLs	**Super Sets** Door Pull Ups & Let Me Ins, Let Me Ins w/ 4-6 second pause at top & Let Me Ups, Let Me Ups w/reverse grip and feet elevated & Let Me Ins w/palms up	**Interval Sets** Leg Lifts w/hands on chest, Supermans, Bicycles, Hyperextensions w/hands under chin	**Stappers** 6 Let Me Ups w/knees bent, 12 Alternating Side Lunges, 8 Push Ups
Week 9	**Interval Sets** Push Ups w/feet elevated, Chinese Push Ups w/hands elevated, Close Grip Push Ups w/hands elevated, Assisted Dips	**Tabatas** Iron Mikes, Side Jumps, Squats	**Ladders** Let Me Ups, Let Me Ins, Let Me Ups w/reverse grip, Let Me Ins w/palms up	**Super Sets** Hanging Leg Lifts w/knees bent & Iron Crosses, Alternating 1-Legged Hip Extensions & Supermans, V-Ups & Russian Twists	**Stappers** 6 Let Me Ups w/knees bent, 12 Alternating Side Lunges, 8 Push Ups

Week 10	Super Sets	Interval Sets	Tabatas	Ladders	Stappers
	Push Ups w/feet elevated and 1-3 second pause at bottom & Shove Offs, Military Press w/feet elevated & Overhead Presses, Close Grip Push Ups w/feet elevated & Assisted Dips	Bulgarian Split Squat w/1-3 second pause at bottom, Side Lunges w/4-6 second pause at bottom, Toyotas w/4-6 seconds at bottom, 1-Legged RDLs on pillow	Let Me Ups, Let Me Ins, Squats	Bicycles, Hyperextensions w/hands under chin, Hello Darlings, Swimmers	6 Let Me Ups w/knees bent, 12 Alternating Side Lunges, 8 Push Ups

Master Class

for Advanced trainees

~Weeks 1 & 2~

Muscular Endurance Block
(Ladders)

	Day 1 Push/Pull	Day 2 Legs/Core	Day 3 Push/Pull	Day 4 Legs/Core
Exercises:	Alternating 1-Arm Push Ups w/hands elevated	Alternating 1-Legged Squats assisted or off a platform	Alternating 1-Arm Push Ups w/hands elevated	Alternating 1-Legged Squats assisted or off a platform
	Assisted Door Pull Ups (use a chair to place your feet on or jump and concentrate on the negative)	Alternating Back Lunges w/4-6 second pause at bottom	Assisted Door Pull Ups (use a chair to place your feet on or jump and concentrate on the negative)	Alternating Side Lunges w/1-3 second pause at bottom
	Military Press w/feet elevated	Hip Extensions	Military Press	Alternating 1-Legged RDLs on pillow
	Let Me Ups	Supermans	Let Me Ins	Iron Crosses w/knees bent

~Weeks 3 & 4~

Strength Block
(Interval Sets)

	Day 1/ Push	Day 2/ Legs	Day 3/ Pull	Day 4/ Core
Exercises:	1-Arm Push Ups w/hands elevated	1-Legged Squats assisted or off a platform	Door Pull Ups	Hanging Leg-raises (bringing legs parallel to ground)
	Dive Bombers	Bulgarian Split Squats w/4-6 second pause at bottom	Let Me Ins w/1-3 second contraction at top	Pillow Humpers
	Military Press w/feet elevated	Side Lunges w/4-6 second pause at bottom	Let Me Ups	V-Ups
	Dips	1-Legged Hip Extensions	Let Me Ups w/reverse grip	Supermans

~Weeks 5 & 6~

Power Block
(Supersets)

	Day 1/ Push	Day 2/ Legs	Day 3/ Pull	Day 4/ Core
Exercises:	1-Arm Push Ups & Bouncing Push Ups	Pistols & Box Jumps	Door Pull Ups & Let Me Ups	Hanging Leg Lifts & Bicycles
	Military Press w/feet elevated & Dive Bombers	Sissy Squats & Iron Mikes	1-arm Let Me Ins & Let Me Ups w/reverse grip	Pillow Humpers & Supermans
	Surface Tricep Extensions & Shove Offs	Ham Sand-wiches & Side Jumps	Let Me Ins w/ reverse grip and 4-6 second pause at top & Towel Curls	V-Ups & Iron Crosses w/knees bent

~Weeks 7-10~

Undulating Block

	Day 1/ Push	Day 2/ Leg	Day 3/ Pull	Day 4/ Core	Day 5
Week 7	**Ladders** 1-Arm Push Ups w/hands on knee-high surface, Dive Bombers, Dips, Seated Dips	**Super Sets** Pistols & Sissy Squats, Box Jumps & Iron Mikes, Ham Sandwiches & Side Jumps	**Interval Sets** Door Pull Ups, Let Me Ins w/1-3 second contraction at top, Let Me Ups, Let Me Ups w/reverse grip	**Tabatas** Side V-Ups (4 sets on each side), Flutter Kicks w/hands on chest, Squats	**Stappers** 12 Assisted Alternating 1-Legged Squats or Box Jumps, 6 Dive Bombers, 8 Let Me Ups
Week 8	**Tabatas** Push Ups, Shove Offs, Squats	**Ladders** Assisted 1-Legged Squats, Sissy Squats, Side Lunges w/1-3 second pause at bottom, Hip Extensions	**Super Sets** Door Pull Ups & Let Me Ups, 1-arm Let Me Ins & Let Me Ups w/reverse grip and feet elevated, Let Me Ins w/reverse grip & Towel Curls	**Interval Sets** Hanging Leg Lifts (bringing straight legs up parallel to ground), Pillow Humpers, V-Ups, Supermans	**Stappers** 12 Assisted Alternating 1-Legged Squats or Box Jumps, 6 Dive Bombers, 8 Let Me Ups

Week 9	Interval Sets	Tabatas	Ladders	Super Sets	Stappers
	1-Arm Push Ups w/hands elevated, Dive Bombers, Military Press w/feet elevated, Dips	Iron Mikes, Side Jumps, Squats	Assisted Door Pull Ups, Let Me Ups, Let Me Ups w/reverse grip, Let Me Ins	Hanging Leg Lifts & Bicycles, Pillow Humpers & Supermans, V-Ups & Iron Crosses w/knees bent	12 Assisted Alternating 1-Legged Squats or Box Jumps, 6 Dive Bombers, 8 Let Me Ups
Week 10	Super Sets	Interval Sets	Tabatas	Ladders	Stappers
	1-Arm Push Ups & Bouncing Push Ups, Military Press w/feet & Dive Bombers, Surface Triceps Extensions & Shove Offs	1-Legged Squats assisted or off a platform, Bulgarian Split Squats w/4-6 second pause at bottom, Side Lunges w/4-6 second pause at bottom, 1-Legged Hip Extensions	Let Me Ups, Let Me Ins, Squats	Side V-Ups w/bent legs, Bam Bams, Leg Lifts w/hands on chest, Hyperextensions w/hands under chin	12 Assisted Alternating 1-Legged Squats or Box Jumps, 6 Dive Bombers, 8 Let Me Ups

Chief Class
for the Elite

~Weeks 1 & 2~

Muscular Endurance Block
(Ladders)

	Day 1 Push/Pull	Day 2 Legs/Core	Day 3 Push/Pull	Day 4 Legs/Core
Exercises:	Alternating 1-Arm Push Ups w/hands elevated	Alternating Pistols	Alternating 1-Arm Push Ups w/hands elevated	Alternating 1-Legged Squats
	Door Pull Ups	Iron Mikes	Door Pull Ups	Box Jumps
	Dive Bombers	Alternating 1-Legged Hip Extensions	Military Press w/feet elevated	Sissy Squats
	Let Me Ups w/feet elevated	Pillow Humpers	Alternating 1-Arm Let Me Ins	Iron Crosses

YOU ARE YOUR OWN GYM

~Weeks 3 & 4~

Strength Block
(Interval Sets)

	Day 1/ Push	Day 2/ Legs	Day 3/ Pull	Day 4/ Core
Exercises:	1-Arm Push Ups	Pistols	Door Pull Ups w/ 1-3 second pause at top	Hanging Leg Lifts (all the way up)
	Handstand Push Ups	Bulgarian Split Squat w/ 4-6 second pause at bottom	1-arm Let Me Ins	Pillow Humpers
	Dive Bombers	Sissy Squats	Let Me Ups w/ reverse grip & feet elevated	Jack Knives
	Surface Triceps Extensions w/ about hip height surface	Iron Mikes	Let Me Ins w/ 4-6 second contraction at top	Supermans

~Weeks 5 & 6~

Power Block
(Supersets)

	Day 1/ Push	Day 2/ Legs	Day 3/ Pull	Day 4/ Core
Exercises:	1-Arm Push Ups w/feet elevated & Bouncing Push Ups	Alternating Pistols w/1-3 second pause at bottom & Box Jumps	Door Pull Ups w/4-6 second pause at top & Let Me Ups w/ feet elevated	Hanging Leg Lifts w/4-6 pause at top (bringing feet to hands) & slow Bicycles (taking 2 seconds to pull each knee in)
	Handstand Push Ups w/1-3 second pause at Bottom & Dive Bombers	Sissy Squats w/ 1-3 seconds at Bottom & Iron Mikes	1-arm Let Me Ins w/1-3 second contraction at top & Let Me Ups w/reverse grip and feet elevated	Pillow Humpers & Supermans
	Surface Triceps Extensions w/ about knee height surface & Shove Offs	Ham Sandwiches & Side Jumps	Pull Ups (touching sternum) & Let Me Ins w/reverse grip and 4-6 second contraction at top	Jack Knives & Iron Crosses

YOU ARE YOUR OWN GYM

Undulating Block

	Day 1/ Push	Day 2/ Leg	Day 3/ Pull	Day 4/ Core	Day 5
Week 7	**Ladders** 1-Arm Push Ups, Handstand Push Ups, Dive Bombers, Dips w/1-3 second pause at bottom	**Super Sets** Alternating Pistols w/1-3 second pause at bottom & Box Jumps, Sissy Squats w/1-3 second pause at bottom & Iron Mikes, Ham Sandwiches (without using hands) & Side Jumps	**Interval Sets** Door Pull Ups w/1-3 second pause at top, 1-arm Let Me Ins, Let Me Ups w/reverse grip & feet elevated, Let Me Ins w/reverse grip 4-6 second contraction at top	**Tabatas** V-Ups, Side-V-Ups (Alternating sides after each set for a total of 4 sets on each side), Mountain Climbers, Squats	**Stappers** 12 Alternating Pistols (6 total on each side) or 24 Iron Mikes (jumping as high as possible), 6 Handstand Push Ups, 8 Door Pull Ups

Week 8	Tabatas	Ladders	Super Sets	Interval Sets	Stappers
	Push Ups, Shove Offs, Mountain Climbers, Burpees	1-Legged Squats, Sissy Squats, Iron Mikes, 1-Legged Hip Extensions	Door Pull Ups w/4-6 second pause at top & Let Me Ups w/feet elevated, 1-arm Let Me Ins w/1-3 second contraction at top & Let Me Ups w/reverse grip and feet elevated, Pull Ups (touching sternum) & Let Me Ins w/reverse grip and 4-6 second contraction at top	Hanging Leg Lifts (all the way up), Pillow Humpers, Jack Knives, Supermans	12 Alternating Pistols or 24 Iron Mikes (jumping as high as possible), 6 Handstand Push Ups, 8 Door Pull Ups

Week 9	Interval Sets	Tabatas	Ladders	Super Sets	Stappers
	1-Arm Push Ups, Handstand Push Ups, Dive Bombers, Surface Triceps Extensions w/ about hip height surface	Iron Mikes, Side Jumps, Squat Thrusts, Squats	Door Pull Ups, Let Me Ups, Let Me Ups w/reverse grip, Alternating 1-arm Let Me ins	Hanging Leg Lifts (bringing feet to hands) w/4-6 second pause at top & Bicycles (12 slowly on each side for 24 total), Pillow Humpers & Supermans, Jack Knives & Iron Crosses (6 slow on each side for 12 total)	12 Alternating Pistols or 24 Iron Mikes, 6 Handstand Push Ups, 8 Door Pull Ups
Week 10	Super Sets	Interval Sets	Tabatas	Ladders	Stappers
	1-Arm Push Ups w/feet elevated & Bouncing Push Ups, Handstand Push Ups & Dive Bombers w/pauses when your chest is between your hands on the concentric portion of the movement, Surface Tricep Extensions w/ about knee height surface & Shove Offs	1-Legged Squats, Bulgarian Split Squat w/overhead backpack press at bottom, Iron Mikes, Ham Sandwiches	Assisted Door Pull Ups (use a chair to place your feet on or jump and concentrate on the negative), Let Me Ups, Let Me Ins, Mountain Climbers	Jack Knives, Pillow Humpers, Alternating Side V-Ups w/legs straight, Supermans	12 Alternating Pistols or 24 Iron Mikes, 6 Handstand Push Ups, 8 Door Pull Ups

Appendix 1.

Household Equipment

As you've seen, with enough keen observation and creativity, you can transform just about any room into a total body fitness center. And, although it is not necessary for my programs, you'd be surprised at how much resistance equipment you can create from basic household items, replacing the need for dumbbells in traditional strength exercises.

Take bicep curls for example. Just because you don't have dumbbells doesn't mean you can't do them. You can use gallon jugs of water (filled to your appropriate level), grocery bags filled with things, or my favorite whether I'm at home or in another country: A duffel bag or backpack filled with books, magazines, newspapers, cans of food, rocks, sand, and/or recycled full water bottles. Add things to the backpack until you have the perfect weight and hold the top strap. You can even make a proper handle out of it: Just brake off a few inches of a stick or branch that's the proper width for a handle and use tape to fasten it to the backpack's top handle. Most backpacks can easily hold up to 60 pounds, some a lot more.

You can use backpacks in place of dumbbells for myriad movements like shoulder raises, tricep exercises, or upright rows. Throw it on your back to increase the resistance to any Pull Up, Squat, Lunge, you name it. Or give your child a piggyback during leg exercises, or even your girlfriend or your wife (though not both at the same time—that could be trouble).

Books—telephone books, text books, encyclopedias, a dictionary—can also be utilized, as can bricks and soup cans, not to mention the things you can alter the weight of. Wearing a backpack full of rocks and holding a five gallon bucket filled with water adds some serious intensity to my Calf Raises. Sandbags can be put on your knees for Sitting Calf Raises.

With a rope, or any kind of long strap, you can do Let Me In's by looping it around a tree, fence or railing, using one or both hands. If you want to buy olympic rings with straps these are great too. The options are nearly endless. Just look around you and get creative. Chances are you already have all the equipment you'll ever need.

Just a few of the many ways to make equipment out of household items.

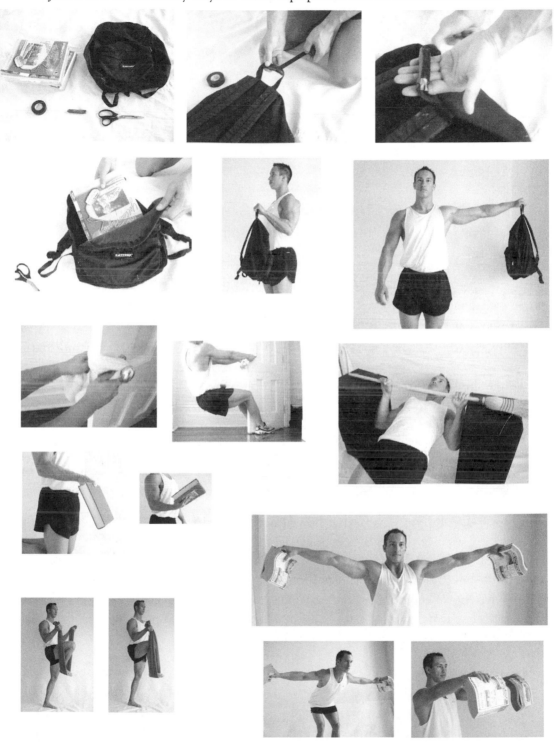

Appendix 2.   The 6 Necessary Training Principles behind Any Successful Program

CONSISTENCY: Truly the gatekeeper to long-term success. We need to be consistent with a good training program, diet, and adequate rest. Not consistent for two months, I mean consistent for years, even decades. If you fall off the horse, get back on. Sound training principles must be a way of life.

RECOVERY: Is there adequate rest built into the program, or will it cause you to over-train? (See the *More is Better* myth for signs and symptoms of overtraining.)

REGULARITY: The body thrives on regularity. A program shouldn't consist of random exercises performed at random intervals, with random intensity and random repetitions. As my Air Traffic Control Instructor used to say, "We need a system and then a plan—that's when we're dangerous." The body won't adapt to random activity. Without regularity, there is nothing to adapt to. It is best to set goals and regularly and methodically do those exercises that get us there fastest.

VARIETY: Variety doesn't mean different exercises every time we workout. We can do the same few exercises for each body part for years. What needs to vary is the intensity, volume, and rest between sets. In order to adjust intensity using bodyweight exercises, different variations of the same movements and different types of workouts need to be performed.

PROGRESSION: It's amazing how much this principle is overlooked in gyms across the nation. I used to see it all the time, people going to the gym year after year, lifting the exact same weight. Why? Considering the other principles are in place, probably because they don't have a program that progresses from easier to more difficult movements, whether it's more weight, a harder variation, more reps, less rest between sets, faster tempo (more reps/less time), or any combination of these. At the same time, it is also possible that a program progresses too rapidly, causing over-training.

OVERLOAD: In order to change body composition and gain strength we need to put muscles under stress that they are unaccustomed to. The body requires new stimulus to force it to adapt. Then, when the adaptation has occurred, once again new stimulus beyond what was previously done is required. Progression and overload go hand-in-hand, and the right amount of each is essential.

Appendix 3.

The Science behind the Program

PERIODIZATION: The Backbone to the Ultimate Strength Program

Knowing why and how you should be doing each workout, rather than blindly going through the motions, will give you the drive to push through hard times, prevent burnout, and give you the know-how to customize the program as your body changes and adapts. The key ingredient to my program is **periodization**: Structured fluctuation of training volume and intensity.

Training Volume: Number of sets multiplied by number of reps.

Training Intensity: Difficulty of a movement. For example, a One-Arm Push Up has a higher intensity than a Classic Push Up.

Variety, regularity, specificity, progression, overload, and recovery—the 6 necessary training principles—are affected by periodically switching from high-volume, low-intensity training to low-volume, high-intensity training. Simply put, a program should transition from a lot of relatively easy work to a smaller amount of more difficult work. This increases athletic performance while avoiding common pitfalls such as overtraining and injury. Myriad studies have demonstrated that periodized programs yield greater changes in strength and body composition than non-periodized programs that consist of little or no fluctuation in volume and intensity, like those of so many other books.

In a periodized program, particular skills—muscular endurance, strength, and power—are emphasized for set periods of time called "blocks." Typically, **muscular endurance** is trained during the *high-volume/low-intensity* (HVLI) block, which is where my program uses "ladders" instead of rigid numbers of sets and reps. **Strength** is trained during a *medium-volume/medium-intensity* block with sets in the 6 - 12 rep range. Finally, **power** is trained during the *low-volume/high-intensity* (LVHI) block with sets in the 1 - 5 rep range. The blocks progress from HVLI to LVHI by decreasing the number of reps and/or sets (volume) while increasing the amount of resistance or the difficulty of movements (intensity).

Simple enough, right? *Heh, heh...* Well, it gets better, because there are different types of periodization, and each of the two primary methods has pros and cons depending on the fitness level of the individual. Because of this, my program utilizes both linear periodization and undulating periodization, which are explained below. Please don't get exasperated over the names of these cycles. You'll be amazed at their simplicity.

Linear Periodization (LP) is the traditional and most popular of periodizing programs. LP progresses from HVLI to LVHI in a linear fashion in 2 - 4 week blocks.

As the total number of reps decrease and the difficulty of movements increase, the emphasis shifts from muscular endurance to strength and then finally to power. The rest intervals between sets should increase along with the intensity as an LP program progresses through the different blocks. Usually, 30 - 60 seconds of rest is taken during the muscular endurance block, 90 - 120 seconds for the strength block, and 2.5 - 5 minutes for the power block.

This method of periodization is good for beginners or those that have had a long time off, because it allows adequate time for joints to adapt to new movements and movement proficiency to develop during a gradual increase in intensity. Jumping right into high-intensity movements is asking for trouble. Additionally, HVLI training gives beginners great results, mainly due to an increase in movement proficiency, while preventing injuries and overtraining. The HVLI block is the time to become familiar with exercises and their variations, giving you a lot of relatively easy practice.

While this method is good for untrained individuals, it has the disadvantage of letting the skills that aren't being trained deteriorate in intermediate or advanced trainees. This is due to the long duration (2 - 4 weeks) of each phase, which emphasizes only one particular skill. It also lacks the variety of other methods, which can lead to boredom.

Daily Undulating Periodization (DUP) trains a different skill each day by daily fluctuating volume and intensity. An HVLI training day that emphasizes muscular endurance might be followed by an LVHI day that emphasizes power, and one that emphasizes strength the next day. This method has a lot of variety—great for keeping your body guessing and your morale high. It also prevents detraining of skills, because each skill is trained weekly. Studies have shown that this type of periodization yields twice the strength gains of the traditional LP method.

Since all skills will be trained each week, beginning with week 1, DUP is only for those with adequate training to perform high-intensity workouts without injuring themselves.

Now for my program.

The first 6 weeks use LP. Muscular endurance, strength and power are trained in 2-week blocks until DUP begins on week 7, and lasts 4 weeks until the end of week 10. By using LP *and* DUP we get the best of both worlds. Beginners are able to reap the benefits of LP's sensible progression and the enhanced gains of DUP. Also, since this is a continuously repeating program, the six weeks of LP help prevent burnout from the four-week DUP block that contains an extra, fifth day of working out and high-intensity interval training (HIIT) which is amazingly effective for building muscle, burning fat, increasing cardiovascular endurance, and strength.

Whether or not you decide to use my program, be sure to incorporate some type of periodization into your training. Any type of periodization is better than none. Going balls to the wall all the time, even at low-volume, is a sure way to over-train and eventually injure yourself. This applies to any type of strength and conditioning training, whether it is weightlifting, running, cycling, rowing, or anything else. Keep in mind that there are endless variations to periodization. The methods that I have selected best suit strength and conditioning training through bodyweight exercises. My program develops all eight fitness skills: Strength, power, speed, muscular and cardiovascular endurance through the manipulation of volume (sets & reps), intensity (difficulty of a movement), and time (work and rest periods); while the remaining skills—balance, coordination, and flexibility—develop by progressing to bodyweight exercises that challenge them to ever increasing degrees.

A percentage of the author's royalties will be donated to the

Special Operations Warrior Foundation,

which provides full scholarships and counseling

to the surviving children of special operations personnel who die

in operational or training missions, and immediate financial assistance

to severely wounded personnel and their families.

www.specialops.org

This book is available at your favorite bookseller

or come see us at MarkLauren.com

to order signed books with free shipping.